J.B. COLLIP AND THE DEVELOPMENT OF
MEDICAL RESEARCH IN CANADA

To Uncle Syd & Aunt Jane,

With best regards.

[signature]

Toronto, Canada

MCGILL-QUEEN'S/ASSOCIATED MEDICAL SERVICES
(HANNAH INSTITUTE) Studies in the History of Medicine,
Health, and Society
Series Editors: S.O. Freedman and J.T.H. Connor

Volumes in this series have financial support from Associated Medical Services,
Inc., through the Hannah Institute for the History of Medicine Program.

J.B. Collip and the Development of Medical Research in Canada

Extracts and Enterprise

ALISON LI

McGill-Queen's University Press

Montreal & Kingston · London · Ithaca

© McGill-Queen's University Press 2003
ISBN 0-7735-2609-9

Legal deposit fourth quarter 2003
Bibliothèque nationale du Québec

Printed in Canada on acid-free paper.

This book has been published with the help of a grant from the Humanities
and Social Sciences Federation of Canada, using funds provided by the
Social Sciences and Humanities Research Council of Canada. Funding has
also been received from the Associated Medical Services, Inc.

McGill-Queen's University Press acknowledges the support of the Canada
Council for the Arts for our publishing program. We also acknowledge the
financial support of the Government of Canada through the Book
Publishing Industry Development Program (BPIDP) for our publishing
activities.

National Library of Canada Cataloguing in Publication

Li, Alison I-Syin, 1963–
    J.B. Collip and the development of medical research in Canada / Alison Li.

(McGill-Queen's / Associated Medical Services [Hannah Institute] studies
in the history of medicine, health, and society; no. 18)
Includes bibliographical references and index.
ISBN 0-7735-2609-9

    1. Collip, J.B. (James Bertram), 1892–1965. 2. Medical scientists – Canada
– Biography. 3. Medicine – Research – Canada – History. I. Title.

R464.C65L4 2003   616.4'62027'092   C2003-902323-0

All photographs reproduced in this book are from J.B. Collip Papers,
MS Collection 269, Scrapbook 1, the Thomas Fisher Rare Book Library,
University of Toronto. They have been published with permission of the
Thomas Fisher Rare Book Library, University of Toronto.

This book was typeset by Dynagram Inc. in 10/12 Sabon.

To my parents

Contents

Acknowledgments

Many people have guided and encouraged me in writing this book. Michael Bliss has been constant in his support and tremendously generous with his knowledge and insight. His own scholarly knowledge of James Bertram Collip has been a great asset to me. Dr Barbara Collip Wyatt and Dr C.J. Wyatt graciously welcomed me into their home in Rome, Georgia, and allowed me to share in their treasured memories of her father.

Sandra McRae and Marianne Ainley steered me towards writing on Collip many years ago and, since then, have remained unfailing in their belief in this project. Terrie Romano has been an invaluable colleague throughout the writing of this book, a sure source of keen judgment, fortitude, and wit. Gordon Baker provided his ruthless editor's eye and steadfast support. Beth Smith, Eric Mills, Jennifer Hubbard, John Swann, and Kelly Fox kindly pointed out important sources of research materials. Relatives and friends, especially my brother, have provided patience, good humour, and warm hospitality during my research trips: Paula and C.P. Wu in Vancouver; Monica and Arthur Loh in New York; Linda, Brian, Jennifer, and Stephanie Cheng in Edmonton; Tim and Mimi Lee in London; and Corinne Lacey in Montreal.

I am indebted to the family and friends of Collip who shared their recollections and insights with me: Dr Charles Beer, Dr Kenneth Carroll, Dr Robert Cleghorn, Dr Robert MacBeth, Dr Abe Neufeld, and Dr A.C. Wallace. I am grateful to have had the opportunity to interview Dr Robert Noble before his death and to have been allowed to copy and transcribe the set of recordings he had made of interviews he conducted with Collip's colleagues in the 1970s.

I would like to thank the archivists and librarians who have facilitated my research: Elaine Challacombe, Wangensteen Historical Library, University of Minnesota; Lorraine Collette, National Research Council Secretariat; J.T.H. Connor, University Hospital Museum, London, Ontario; Edna Hadjnal, Fisher Rare Book Library, University of Toronto; Rob Michel, McGill University Archives; D.C. Mortimer, National Research Council Archives; Ed Phelps, Regional Collection, University of Western Ontario; Henri Pilon, Trinity College Archives; William Roberts, University of California, Berkeley Archives; Ken Stephens, Rare Book Library, Canadian Institute for Scientific and Technical Information; Richard Wolfe, Francis A. Countway Library, Harvard University; and the staff of the University of Alberta Archives and the Library of the American Philosophical Society. Nate Caradarelli provided copies of his two manuscripts on the work of Adolph Hanson. Ayerst Laboratories provided materials from the company history. Thanks also to Phillip Cercone of McGill-Queen's University Press for shepherding this project over several years. I acknowledge the generous support of the Hannah Institute for the History of Medicine (Associated Medical Services) and the Atkinson College Junior Research Fund.

Many other teachers and colleagues have offered me careful criticism and guidance. In particular, I thank Trevor Levere, Pauline Mazumdar, and Jacalyn Duffin. Colleagues, both in and out of the academy, have generously helped me carve out and defend precious hours for writing even when it meant I had fewer to devote to my other responsibilities. My husband, Ernie Hamm, has been a source of astute advice and endless encouragement to me in bringing this project to fruition; his support has been invaluable.

This book is dedicated to my parents, Anita and Pai Lin Li, who have inspired and sustained me in countless ways and whose enthusiastic interest in my work has never flagged.

Introduction

Historical accounts of medical research in Canada almost inevitably begin with a proud reference to the isolation of insulin at the University of Toronto in 1921–22. The insulin discovery, a dramatic triumph of science over dread disease, had powerful repercussions in the lives of those who were touched by it. Diabetics and their doctors suddenly gained a potent tool in treating a deadly condition. The Canadian public was given a vivid demonstration that its medical scientists could rank among the best in the world. The subsequent burst of enthusiasm for medical research brought an infusion of young investigators and funds to the field. In the lives of its four discoverers – Frederick Grant Banting, Charles Herbert Best, John James Rickard Macleod, and James Bertram Collip – insulin wrought irrevocable changes.

Banting, Best, and Collip, all young men at the time of the medical breakthrough, found that the insulin discovery marked them for the rest of their lives. These three Canadians would be regarded as being among the leaders of their country's medical research community for the next several decades. Their careers were given an immeasurable boost because of the prestige they gained as scientific heroes, but they also benefited in a very material sense through their share in the substantial insulin royalties. Perhaps most importantly, they became driven to live up to the mighty legacy of their early success.

Banting and Best are still synonymous with the insulin discovery in the popular mind. Macleod, along with Banting, won the Nobel Prize in recognition of his role. Of the four discoverers, the least known and celebrated is J.B. Collip, the shy, intuitive biochemist who, on a late

January night in 1922, watched the first purified sample of insulin precipitate out of a murky alcohol solution. At that moment, Collip, aged only twenty-nine, stepped into the forefront of Canada's fledgling medical research community.

In the early decades of the twentieth century, medical research in Canada could be pursued only by a select few. By mid-century, it had grown into a systematic, large-scale enterprise involving teams of professional scientists and dozens of laboratories in universities, government, and industry. J.B. Collip, skilled both as a bench scientist and an entrepreneur of science, represents a particularly successful part of this change. His story gives us some insight into the forces that transformed the landscape of Canadian medical research.

Thus far, Collip has received attention from historians only in his connection with specific discoveries or with other figures in the history of medical science. This biography examines his career and his life as a whole.[1] Collip was a member of the first generation of medical researchers to obtain a PhD at a Canadian university and then to pursue a successful research career within the country. His first major achievement was to contribute to the isolation of insulin in 1921–22, the definitive account of which is by Michael Bliss in *The Discovery of Insulin*.[2] Collip later went on to important work on the parathyroid hormone, the placental hormones, and anterior pituitary hormones.

This biography also serves as an exploratory study of the emergence of systematic, institutionalized medical research in Canada. Leaders of the emerging research enterprise during this critical period faced several challenges: how to balance laboratory and clinical interests in determining research programs; how to raise funds for experimental investigation in an era before large-scale government support of medical research; how to respond to the opportunities and demands posed by the commercial development of medical products; and how to adapt the laboratory group to the changing scale and character of experimental work.

Collip's success as a scientist and a scientific entrepreneur lay in how he met these challenges. He concentrated on basic research but remained alert to potential therapeutic applications. He used his entrepreneurial skills to gain funding from private and commercial sources. He collaborated closely with pharmaceutical companies. Finally, he gathered a group of associates and melded their diverse talents and disciplinary training to form an effective scientific team.

The story opens with an examination of the formative influences in Collip's education and early scientific work. Chapter 1 describes the undergraduate and graduate training Collip received at the University of Toronto under the guidance of A.B. Macallum, an early proponent of original investigation in the medical sciences. The chapter continues with a discussion of Collip's early career as a professor at the University of Alberta.

Chapter 2 traces Collip's experiences during the pivotal event in his life, the discovery of insulin. Its focus is on how the discovery affected Collip's broader intellectual and professional development.

Chapter 3 examines the impact of the insulin discovery on Collip's life and work. The chapter continues with a study of a priority dispute that developed over his next major accomplishment, the preparation of an active extract of the parathyroid hormone. This episode reflects the tensions surrounding the professionalization of research in endocrinology and the commercial development of medical products.

Chapter 4 presents an analysis of Collip's role in rebuilding the prestige of McGill University's Faculty of Medicine. It examines his discovery and development of the placental hormone product Emmenin. It elaborates on the theme developed in the previous chapter, that while collaborative ventures with pharmaceutical firms were very important to the support of Collip's research enterprise, they sometimes engendered conflicts with established codes of behaviour in medical research.

The scientific content of Collip's research work during his "great years" is examined in Chapter 5. This chapter describes Collip's activities as the head of a large team of researchers with a variety of disciplinary backgrounds. A fortuitous configuration of personnel in the laboratory provided the set of skills necessary to put Collip's group in the forefront of a very competitive field of research. Collip's venture in developing the theory of antihormones, however, was less successful than his work in manipulative biochemistry.

Chapter 6 focuses on Collip's struggles to establish a research institute. It follows the course of his failed application to the Rockefeller Foundation and his negotiations with administrators at McGill. It concludes with an analysis of the reasons that Collip's research career finally came to an end.

Chapter 7 contains a survey of the work of the National Research Council's Associate Committee on Medical Research (later renamed the Division of Medical Research) during the twenty years that Collip was associated with it. It outlines the manner in which the federal government gradually accepted responsibility for the financial support of medical research and goes on to suggest the ways in which the experiences of Collip's own career are reflected in the policies and practices instituted during these years. The biography concludes with a discussion of the broader implications of this study.

Today, discussions of medical science abound with terms like patents and profits, venture capital, and private sector partnerships. Academic scientists double as biotechnology entrepreneurs. Some might be surprised to know that this is by no means new territory for Canadian medical science and that some of its early pioneers – far from being isolated geniuses in ivy-covered towers – were quite adept at traversing this difficult terrain. Collip's story tells us much about how large-scale, systematic government funding for medical research arose out of a patchwork of public and private funds. Now, half a century later, when the commercialization of university research is the focus of increasing public scrutiny and the guidelines delineating private rights and public responsibilities seem in need of greater clarification, the lessons of this story are more pertinent than ever.

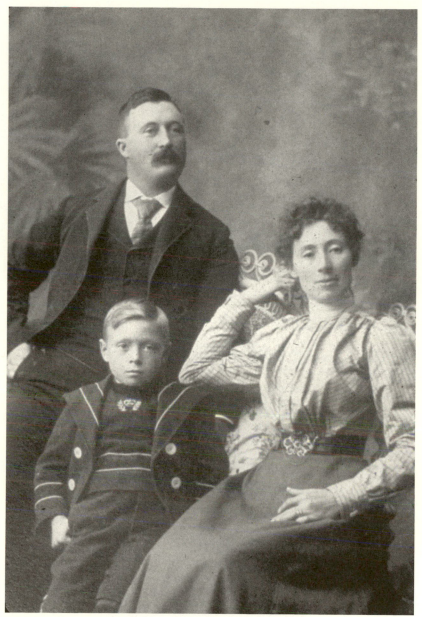

James Bertram Collip with his father (James Denis Collip) and mother (Mahala Frances Vance Collip). Portrait made in Belleville, Ontario, about 1898.

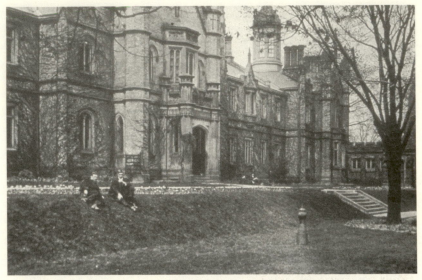

Snapshot of Bert during student days at Trinity College, University of Toronto, about 1912.

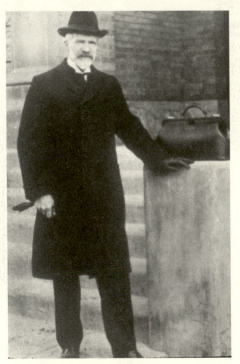

Archibald Macallum, about 1905.

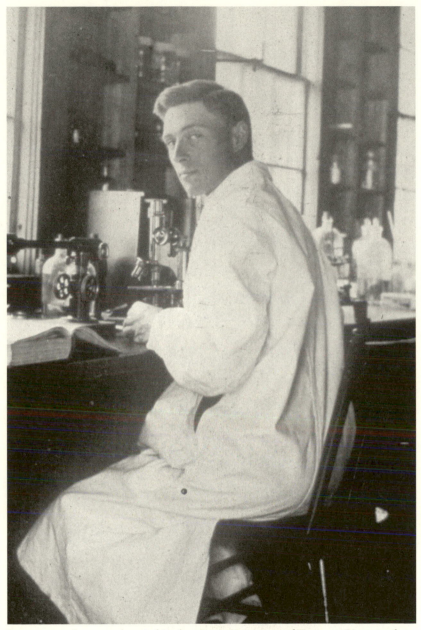

Bert as a graduate student in biochemistry, University of Toronto. Picture taken about 1914–15.

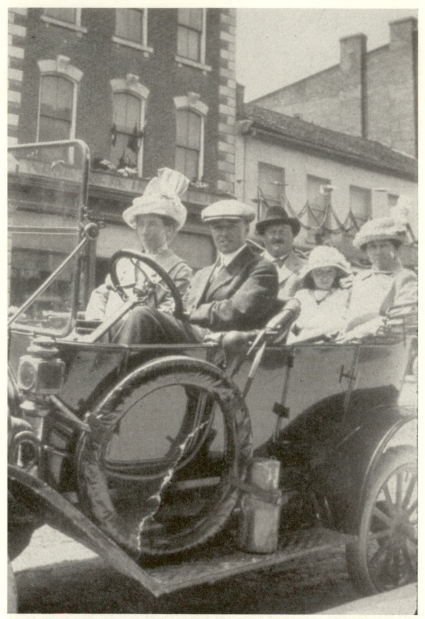

Snapshot of Collip family made in Belleville, Ontario, about 1915. Pictured are Bert Collip (driver) with his mother by his side; in the back seat are his father (James Denis), his sister (Rita), and his aunt (Minnie).

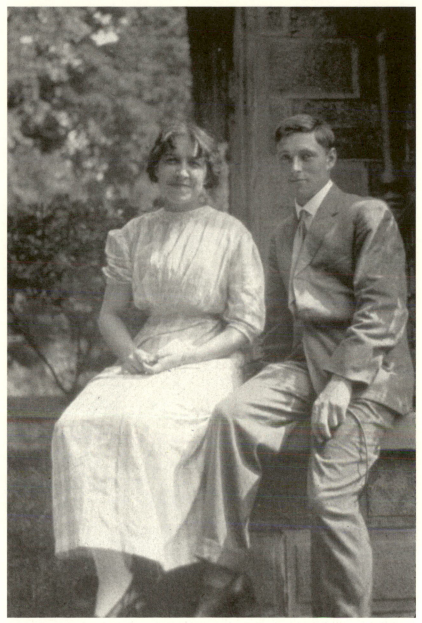

Ray Vivian Ralph and Bert Collip during courtship. Photograph made at the Ralph residence in Dundas, Ontario, probably in the summer of 1915. They were married in this home on 28 December 1915.

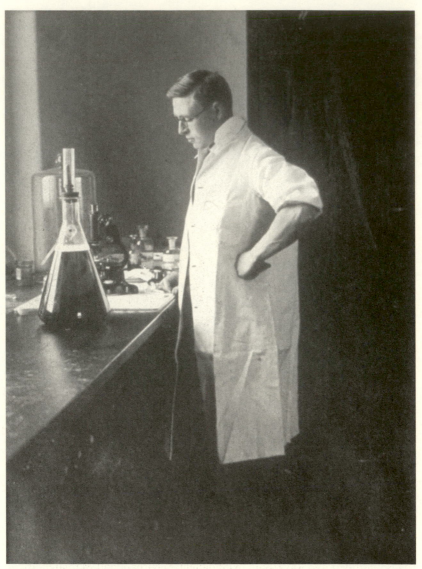

Professor Collip in laboratory at the University of Alberta, Edmonton (about 1927).

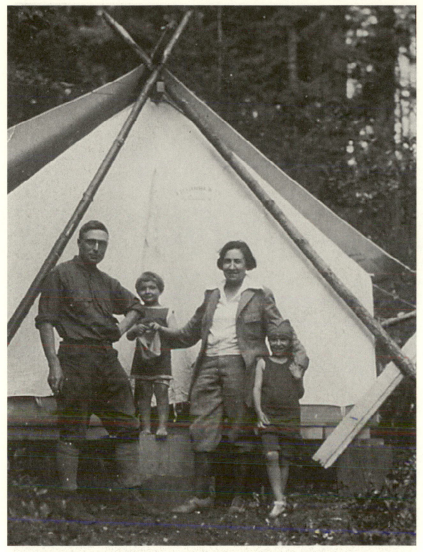

Snapshot of Bert and Ray Collip, with daughters Barbara and Margaret, at Nanaimo, British Columbia, about 1927. Collip worked at the Pacific Biological Station at Nanaimo during several summers while at the University of Alberta.

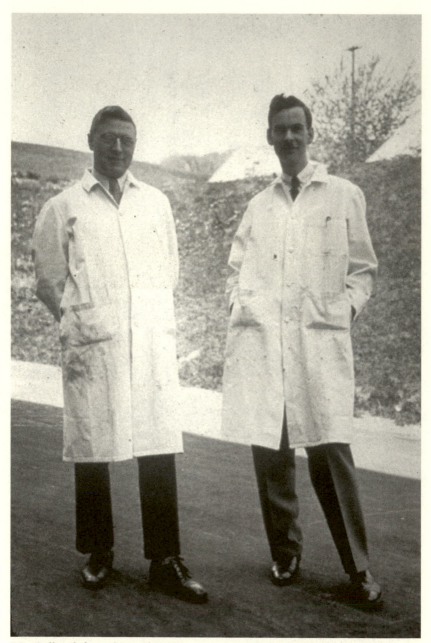

J.B. Collip (left) and David L. Thomson, McGill University, about 1933.

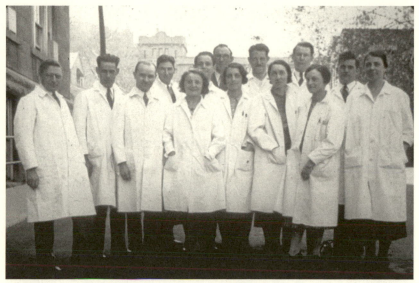

Dr Collip with his laboratory staff at McGill University, Montreal, about 1933. Dr Hans Selye and Dr J.S.L. Brown are in the group. This picture is taken by the side of the Biological Building. Collip's laboratory was then located on the third floor of this building.

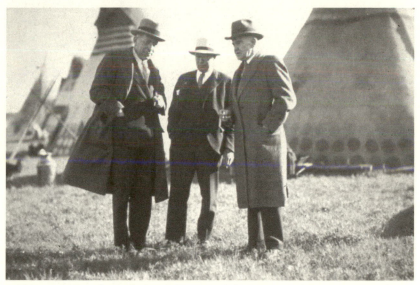

Collip (centre) and Sir Frederick Banting (left). Picture is believed to have been taken in Calgary, probably in 1936, on the way to Vancouver for the Canadian Medical Association Meeting.

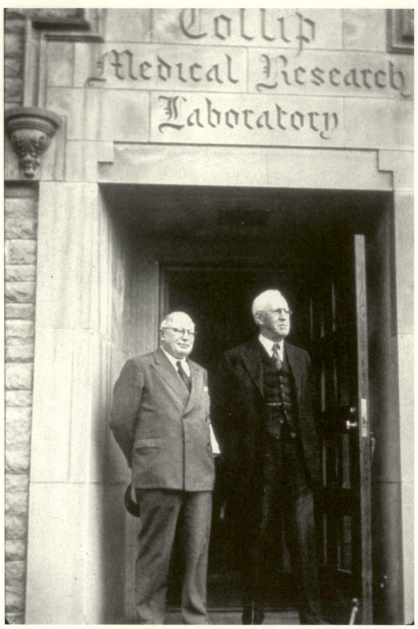

Dr J.B. Collip (left) and Sir Henry Dale at the main entrance of the Collip Building, at the University of Western Ontario, October 1947. Sir Henry was attending the proceedings of the eleventh annual meeting of the Canadian Physiological Society held at the University of Western Ontario Medical School.

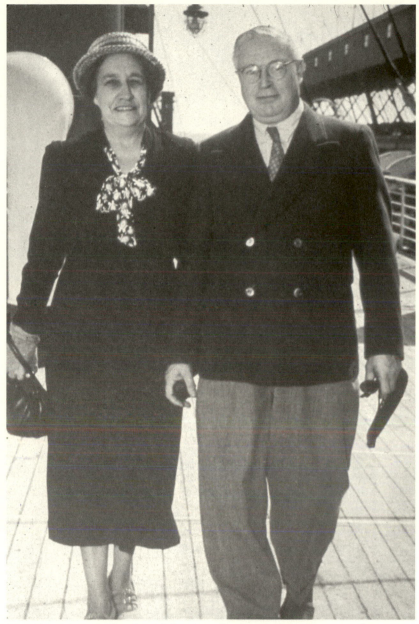

Dr and Mrs J.B. Collip aboard the Canadian Pacific liner *Empress of France* bound for the United Kingdom, August 1949. Collip acted as vice-president of the International Congress of Biochemistry, held at Cambridge, England.

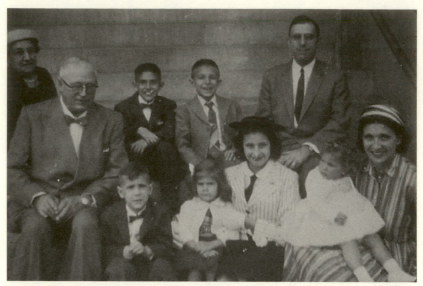

Dr and Mrs Collip with daughter Barbara Wyatt's family, in Rome, Georgia. All sitting on steps of the Episcopal Church after the baptismal service for granddaughter Margaret, 24 February 1957.

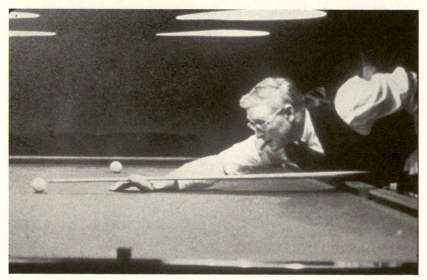

Informal snapshot of Bert enjoying one of his favourite pastimes (billiards), at his home, 622 Sydenham Avenue, Westmount, Quebec, about 1941.

J.B. COLLIP AND THE DEVELOPMENT OF
MEDICAL RESEARCH IN CANADA

I

The Research Ideal, 1892–1920

I do not know whether I am unique in my feelings in this regard but I think it must be a fair assumption that it is the personal satisfaction experienced by the researcher of work accomplished and achievement that keeps him at his task irrespective of position or financial reward. I think it to be most important that the young man or woman undertaking a research career should be imbued very early with the intense if not burning desire to extend the frontiers of knowledge, and this should be his or her paramount thought.

J.B. Collip, July 1948[1]

In the last decade of the nineteenth century, the township of Thurlow, Ontario, hummed with prosperity. It was enviably situated atop fine-quality loam, its landscape undulating and its climate agreeable. The river Moira and its tributaries flowed through the township and then continued a short distance southwest towards the city of Belleville, itself located midway on the main route between Toronto and Montreal. A century before, the area had become home to United Empire Loyalists seeking refuge in British North America after the American Revolution. An enterprising loyalist captain had set up the first saw and grist mills in the area, and the small settlement had soon become a trading centre for a burgeoning lumber industry. By the time the lumber trade had begun to fail in the 1870s, discoveries of mineral troves in the north brought new money through town. The Grand Trunk Railway and a regular steamship service helped to transport the bounty of this area – its timber, limestone, and a variety of agricultural products – to other parts of the world while bringing back more and more hopeful newcomers.[2]

Englishman James Coe Collip was one of many immigrants drawn to Belleville. He married Ellen Mullens and in 1873 started a market garden in the first concession of Thurlow Township, just outside the city. His son, James Denis Collip, grew up working alongside his father, gaining, according to the local paper, "a thorough knowledge of everything pertaining to plant life."[3] Thus, in his time, the younger Collip was able to build a thriving business. He married Mahala Frances Vance, a schoolteacher and a woman remarked upon for her determination and self-reliance. On 20 November 1892 their first child, a son, was born. He was named James Bertram Collip but was known throughout his life as Bert. Bert was raised alone until he was eight years old, when his sister, Rita Emily, was born. The age gap between the siblings meant that Bert and Rita grew up almost like single children.

We know little about Bert's early years. Only snippets can be drawn from family stories and photo albums. During his youth, Bert often earned money by selling his grandfather's produce from a horse and cart. He is recalled as saying, "The last year before I went to college I sold cabbages."[4] We know he attended a one-room country schoolhouse within walking distance of his home and that later he went to Belleville High School.

By the time Bert had reached high school age, his father had become one of the principal florists in the area. The elder Collip had a salesroom at 265 Front Street, Belleville's main business thoroughfare, and two greenhouses in the second concession of Thurlow. According to Belleville's daily newspaper, he had a thriving trade in wholesale and retail, supplying flowers and plants – with "all the latest ideas and designs" – throughout the area and surrounding districts. His greenhouses were "equipped with every convenience for raising all manner of flowers and bedding plants," and he employed several workers and a travelling salesman.[5] The family's comfortable situation is suggested by a photograph of the teenaged Bert proudly posing at the wheel of a fine car, lean and boyishly handsome. This picture is a wonderful presage of Collip's legendary and lifelong love of the automobile.

Bert showed no inclination towards the work of his father and grandfather; instead, he developed an interest in chemistry and a desire to go to university. This ambition was further fanned by a visit from the provost of Trinity College, Toronto. Trinity College was an Anglican institution that had only recently federated with the University of Toronto. As the Collip family belonged to the Anglican Church, Trinity was deemed an appropriate place for Bert's higher education. In 1908, at the tender age of fifteen, Bert Collip matriculated and entered the University of Toronto. His mother was immensely proud of him and would tell her grandchildren in later years how much she had taught him as a child, how quick he had been to learn, and how he had put on his first pair of long pants to go off to university.

Collip seems to have been all too happy to leave Belleville. He would come to refer to his early days as his "life in the country," and even in his later years, he would be known for his aversion to rural living.[6]

TRINITY COLLEGE

The Trinity College that greeted Bert Collip was a bastion of Anglican tradition. Founded in 1852 by the bishop of Toronto, John Strachan, it had remained a staunchly Anglican institution in the years since then. The college was built on Queen Street, west of the city, in order to keep its students safe from dangerous urban influences. By the time Collip arrived at its venerable gates, Trinity had just survived a period of considerable upheaval. The college had given in to the financial realities of the new era and had agreed to surrender its independence in order to federate with the University of Toronto. The university was situated in the city, at Queen's Park, some two miles north and east Trinity's location. Plans for moving the college to the downtown campus were slow to gel, however, and so Trinity would, at least in a physical sense, remain in splendid isolation for another two decades.

In the fifty years since Trinity had been built, the city had crept up to the edges of its grounds. Queen Street bustled with the clop-clop of horse-drawn streetcars taking people to and from the nearby asylum, undertaker's parlour, and candy factory. Pedestrians browsed in foreign-language news shops and conducted their business in the long row of red-brick stores. On the north side of the street stood Trinity's imposing iron gate, beyond which stretched a broad parkland. An elm-lined road led to the main college building, in massive yellow stone, graced by gothic spires carved in the Oxford style. During the summer, Trinity men in sharp whites played cricket on its lawns or lolled in the shady ravine to the east.

Most of the college men came from out of town and almost all resided within Trinity's gates. Trinity took great pride in retaining its academic traditions long after the other colleges had discarded them. Students were expected to wear academic gowns to their lectures during the day and to put on blazers in the evenings. A white surplice was added for chapel each morning. Attendance at chapel was compulsory for students and dons alike, and those who failed to appear could expect to find their names publicly displayed or even to receive a personal note from the provost. It was rumoured that sleepy-eyed men sometimes managed to make it to matins on time only by compromising their attire. The provost found it necessary to issue a note formally forbidding the wearing of pyjamas and slippers under one's gown.

The college buildings were resolutely Victorian, their dusky stone corridors flickering with gaslight. Collip roomed in the upper corridor of the East Wing with divinity student Harding Priest. Each of the residential halls had a nickname, and theirs was known as the Angel's Roost for its preponderance of theology students. In contrast, the lower floors of the wing were famed for the sport of bottle rolling. Its denizens delighted in tossing bottles from either end of a long corridor, with the objective of creating the most explosive collision possible. Collip and Priest shared the typical student accommodations, a small study attached to a tiny room for sleeping, dubbed "the coffin." The rooms were heated by an open-grate fire, the coal for which was charged to the students' accounts. Frugal undergraduates would often forgo lighting their fires until teatime and thus would have to begin their winter mornings by cracking through the ice crusts formed on their wash basins. Many a passionate discussion was held before the grate, with faces deliciously warm and backs icy cold.

When Trinity federated with the University of Toronto, it gave up its degree-granting status for all subjects but divinity. Many courses could be given at the Queen Street location, but those requiring modern laboratory facilities were given at Queen's Park only. Science students from Trinity took most of their courses at the main university, spending hours each week riding the streetcars along Queen and then up McCaul.

Bert blossomed at Trinity. While generally a shy person, he gamely took part in many college activities. He competed in the tennis tournaments and ran in the annual steeplechase on Saints Simon and Jude's day. When the college literary society – "the Lit" – held a mock trial, he took the role of "Dr Collip" and examined the "witnesses" for signs of insanity. When Trinity undergraduates held their annual secret Episkopon ritual, Collip joined in. In this ceremony, the "spirit" of the venerable Father Episkopon would be summoned to the Dining Hall where he would mete out public censures for supposed faults. As Bert's interest in science grew, he found a niche among like-minded students. He founded the Trinity Science Club in 1911 with David Keys and F.M. Turner. During its early years, the club had difficulty competing with the more established societies, such as the Lit and the Glee Club, but a small and active group of supporters persevered. They gathered monthly in rooms of members to learn about recent scientific findings or to have more broadly philosophical discussions about the place of science in the world. In those early years, they heard papers such as "The Relation of Science to Literature" and "The New Gas x-3 Discovered by Professor J.J. Thomson" and debated questions such as "Resolved that the study of science has no other justification than the advancement of human welfare."[7]

In academic work, Collip also flourished. Bert had intended to study medicine when he had first arrived in Toronto but found that, at fifteen, he was too young to enter the medical course. Instead, he enrolled in the honours biochemistry and physiology program. In doing so, he entered into a course of study that had few equivalents in North America. This program had been established in 1904 as a way of creating an elite stream of medical students trained in methods of scientific research. While high school graduates could enter medicine directly, students in the "B and P" program first earned an honours BSc in four years, then completed two further years of study that also served as the first two years of medical training. The program was the legacy of Robert Ramsay Wright and Archibald Byron Macallum, professors at the University of Toronto. Historian Sandra McRae credits Wright and Macallum with bringing the research ideals of biology to the study of medicine and building one of the most progressive pre-clinical programs in North America. The excellent undergraduate honours program, McRae argues, rivalled graduate programs in the United States in its rigorous training in original investigation. In 1909 Abraham Flexner rated the laboratory facilities as being "among the best on the continent."[8]

Ramsay Wright was the chair of natural history and later of the Department of Biology. In the 1880s he built up an active research program and cultivated a group of young research associates. Many of the graduates of the Toronto program went on to become leaders in biological medicine in the United States, including Lewellys Barker, Thomas Cullen, Thomas Futcher, William MacCallum, John B. MacCallum, Robert Russell Bensley, Frank Lillie, Ralph Lillie, and Maud Menten.

A.B. Macallum was among those who studied biology under Wright. He went on to take a PhD at the Johns Hopkins University under the physiologist Henry Newell Martin. When he returned to Canada, he became one of the first to make a career of experimental research in biology, inspiring many of his own students to follow his example.

Macallum developed an active research program in general physiology and general biochemistry. His studies were oriented towards evolutionary questions and the application of chemistry to biological problems. He was particularly concerned with fundamental processes such as growth, energy transformation, and biochemical control. Macallum investigated the operation of these processes in a wide variety of life forms, preferring not to restrict himself to the special problems of human physiology and pathology. In the 1890s he and his associate, Robert Russell Bensley, adapted chemical methods of analysis for use with the microscope. These microchemical techniques allowed them to determine the location of iron, phosphorus, and other materials in tissues and within cells.

Wright and Macallum had both been active in opening the marine biological station of the Biological Board of Canada in 1898. This gave them access to marine organisms for research purposes, a fact that would shape Macallum's work. One line of research that he pursued throughout his career was based on his early investigations of the concentration of various salts in the bodily fluids of jellyfish. His observations led him to speculate that the plasma of animals and plants reflected the composition of the ancient oceans from which life had first emerged; that is, that even after organisms emerged from the seas, they continued to bathe their cells in a solution resembling that in which they had evolved. He regarded plasma as a sort of living fossil record. In the first decade of the twentieth century, Macallum also pursued the question of how surface tension related to the active transport of solutes across membranes. Macallum served as lecturer in biology from 1883 and then as professor of physiology after 1890.

In 1908, the year Collip arrived in Toronto, the chair of physiology was split and Macallum was made the first professor of biochemistry in Canada. Collip had the good fortune to become associated with Macallum at this time. It must have been a heady experience for the young man, coming from his country school, to enter this flourishing intellectual environment where research was promoted with such zeal. Bert did well in his studies and in 1912 graduated at the top of his class. Macallum's message of the research ideal fell on fertile soil with this student as it had with many others. Inspired, Collip decided to give up his plans for medicine and pursue graduate studies instead.

ABSORBING THE RESEARCH IDEAL

The University of Toronto had established the first doctoral program in Canada in 1897. McGill followed with its doctoral program only in 1906. While Macallum was very successful in developing a strong, research-oriented undergraduate honours program, he was less successful in promoting graduate work. It was not until the 1920s, after he had left Toronto, that a fully active graduate program was established. During his tenure, only three students completed PhD programs, one of whom was Collip.

Through these years, Collip's studies were not the sole source of his inspiration. During his final undergraduate year, he began to notice a certain contralto in the Trinity chapel choir. When it became clear that Collip was too shy to act on his own behalf, a classmate intervened and arranged a first meeting with Ray Vivian Ralph. Ray Ralph was the daughter of a druggist from Dundas, Ontario, and an arts student at Trinity's sister college, St Hilda's. Vibrant and fun loving, known to her family as a tomboy, Ray was said to be the one to climb through windows to visit Bert.[9]

Collip continued as a resident at Trinity while doing his graduate work. He was offered a teaching fellowship under Macallum, and this he accepted promptly, entering into the work with great enthusiasm. He absorbed all that Macallum had to teach him. An indefatigable worker, Macallum taught his classes during the day and worked on his research late into the night. Collip later recalled, "I was completely over-awed by the austere and heavily bearded professor, whom I held in great esteem and almost reverence."[10] Macallum's training style consisted of setting problems for investigation and then letting the students work them out for themselves. Collip later grew to appreciate this approach when he ran his own laboratory in much the same way. He quickly learned that Macallum customarily looked in at the laboratory between eleven and twelve at night, and as an eager young student, Collip made sure to be present at that time so as to make a good impression. Before long, he also came to recognize that the quiet hours of the late evenings and weekends were the most productive for laboratory work. Out of this realization sprang his lifelong habit of working all hours of the night.

Collip's research projects were heavily influenced by Macallum's interests in microchemistry and the chemical composition of bodily fluids. Macallum first assigned him to study the microchemistry of the nerve cells of the central ganglionic chain of the medicinal leech. In order to conduct this work, Collip had to make fresh preparations of leech to examine under the ultramicroscope. He acquired some considerable skill in handling the instrument for studies and for taking photomicrographs.

As a beginner in the lab, Collip experienced a couple of mishaps. First, his supply of leeches escaped when he tied the muslin top on their container too loosely. Because he viewed his professor with such awe, Collip hid his mistake and bought a fresh lot of leeches with money from his own pocket. Later, more seriously, he broke the quartz cover slip of the special chamber that was designed for use with the cardioid condenser of the Zeiss ultramicroscope. Again he replaced this at his own expense, even though the cover slip had to be ordered from the German manufacturer. Fortunately, Collip's fear of Macallum faded over time and he began to feel more certain that there was a kind, sympathetic soul behind the severe face.

Collip learned to operate the freezing microtome to prepare sections of the fresh nerve cell material, and then to use the microchemical staining techniques that Macallum had developed to locate chemical components. Frozen sections of the freshly dissected ganglia were dropped on the surface of a chilled solution of silver nitrate. Then the section was transferred to a microscopic slide, mounted in glycerin, and exposed to sunlight. This delicate work required that the tissue be frozen instantaneously and put on the surface of the reagent while still frozen. Usually, this meant that the investigator had to wait for the arrival of winter and, when the mercury dropped sufficiently, prop open a lab window and perform the procedure standing in front of it. Collip conceived an innovative way around this slow and uncertain process, constructing an asbestos-lined box with a plate glass cover and two arm holes with padded sleeves. He used a carbon dioxide jet to chill the air inside the box and then manipulated the microtome through the sleeves. Using his apparatus, Collip was able to find that an intense black staining occurred in the central core of the ganglia and the clusters of nerve cells when the solution reacted with sunlight.

On his visits to the lab, Macallum inspected the young man's progress and generally murmured "very interesting" or "keep at it." The first time he saw the black staining of the ganglia, however, he became tremendously excited and gathered several other professors to see the material. The silver nitrate reaction, he thought, might indicate the presence of adrenalin in the cells. Collip was delighted by Macallum's interest and thrilled at the possible significance of the work. Macallum's enthusiasm was positively infectious.

The possibility that invertebrate nerve cells might contain adrenalin was exciting, but the evidence that Collip was able to summon was only suggestive. The standard test for the presence of adrenalin involved evaluating the effect of a test sample on the blood pressure of dogs. When these tests were done, the results were negative. It was only later that other investigators, using more sensitive methods, would succeed in demonstrating the presence of adrenalin. Collip wrote up his work as a thesis entitled "Some Observations on the Structure and Microchemistry of Nerve Cells." This earned him a master of arts degree in 1913. He also had the honour of having his research incorporated into a joint paper that Macallum presented at the meeting of the International Medical Association and the British Association for the Advancement of Science in Birmingham.[11]

Collip launched into his doctoral work with a new problem assigned to him by Macallum. He was to make a comparative study of the secretion of hydrochloric acid by the gastric tubules of the vertebrate stomach. In this work, as with the previous, Collip was highly influenced by his professor's advocacy of biochemical methods to examine the functional rather than the morphological aspects of tissues. Collip used microchemical methods to localize chemical compounds in the gastric tissue of various species of mammals, birds, reptiles, and amphibians and used this data to theorize about the mechanism that caused the formation of hydrochloric acid in the stomach. He earned his PhD in biochemistry in 1916 for this work, and his thesis was published as a monograph in 1920.[12]

COLLEGE LIFE

Outside the laboratory, Collip thrashed out his ideas about the broader meaning of science with his fellow students at Trinity. He wrote an article for the *Trinity University Review*, the literary journal of the college, entitled, "Mind and the Cerebral Mechanism." He explained the significance of recent scientific findings on the activities of the brain and argued that physiologists, embryologists, and histologists were throwing much light on the question of cognition. Like Macallum, he did not accept vitalist explanations of nature. Yet he also rejected the extreme materialist view that the individual was just a puppet, merely a bundle of reflexes reacting to external stimuli, or that "consciousness is an epiphenomenon." Rather, he argued that the physiologist was only able to study the behaviour of the animal machine and that an explanation of the will or ego behind the behaviour remained outside the bounds of science.[13]

Collip's interests were highly influenced by the evolutionary orientation of his teacher. One paper he read to the Science Club, entitled "Evolution," dealt with the Weismann germ-plasm theory. Another paper was a review of Macallum's theory that the proportions of elements in blood plasma resembled those in the sea water from which the first life forms emerged. Collip's friend and roommate, divinity student Harding Priest, presented a paper to the Theological Society on "Evolution and Christianity." Priest attempted to reconcile evolutionary theory with Christian thought and used the argument from design to suggest that the case for theism was strengthened by the scientific evidence for evolution. In the discussion, Collip suggested "that the idea of law as developed from evolution should be of supreme value for the theologian, as it was for the scientist."[14]

During these years, he continued to court Ray Ralph. A pair of photos from this period show Bert and Ray together with Ray's sister Maude and her fiancé, Reg Turnbull, a divinity student at Knox College. In the first snapshot, the two couples swing happily in a hammock, posing for the photographer in their summer whites. In the second, the four are collapsed in a merry heap on the ground, the hammock crumpled beneath them. Bert and Ray were to marry later that year, just after Christmas, and Maude and Reg would be married three weeks after that.[15]

These happy antics were the last of an era about to pass. Many a typical Trinity student was away at the family cottage in August of 1914 when a fateful newspaper arrived announcing the outbreak of war. By the time students returned to class in the autumn, many Trinity men had already enlisted. The lectures continued, but outside the windows the footfall of officers in training drummed in the distance. Soon the stone corridors emptied of their usual crush of inhabitants. Only a few men and the St Hilda's women remained to fill the class rolls.

Collip pressed on with his research. Around this time, he was introduced to Herber H. Moshier, the first professor of physiology at the University of Alberta. Moshier was a young medical practitioner who had been the second appointment to the Faculty of Medicine at Alberta. An active, vibrant man, he not only taught physiology, pathology, and clinical medicine, but also organized the Student Medical Service, where he provided treatment to students.[16] Moshier invited Collip to join him in Edmonton as a lecturer in biochemistry. In September 1915 Collip took up the appointment, having almost finished his doctorate.

IMBIBING THE WESTERN SPIRIT: THE UNIVERSITY OF ALBERTA

Collip's first job was at a very young institution. The province of Alberta had only been created in 1908, and the provincial university three years later. Edmonton was, as at least one faculty member thought, "a remote backwater of the British Empire." University president Henry Marshall Tory took on the challenge of building an institution of higher learning from scratch. He championed the building of professional faculties so that Albertans could be trained without having to travel to universities in central Canada. The Faculty of Medicine was founded shortly after, in 1913, against some opposition from members of the local medical profession who believed such a venture overly ambitious and likely to result in a second-rate institution. Their children were usually sent East to their own alma maters, McGill or Toronto. Since the University of Alberta medical school was the only one in Canada west of Winnipeg, Manitoba, it had an important position in providing medical teaching and service throughout the West. Tory strongly agreed with the view of Abraham Flexner in his report on medical education of 1910, particularly Flexner's insistence that medical training be founded on the basic sciences and that scholarly research should be promoted. In its early years, the school had only a three-year medical program, which meant that the students had to complete their basic science studies in Alberta, then go east to the medical schools in central Canada to complete their clinical years of training.[17]

Edmonton was located on a high flat plain through which the North Saskatchewan River had carved a sharp groove with two hundred–foot banks. The town had once served as the gateway to Klondike gold. The large majority of Albertans lived in rural settings, many of them new immigrants from Eastern Europe, and newcomers mixed with Native people, Métis, and earlier Anglo-Saxon pioneers. The university was built on the south side of the river, just outside Edmonton, about a mile west of the town of Strathcona, a settlement clustered around the end of the Canadian Pacific Railway's spur line from Calgary. In the early years, students had to march to the outskirts of town and scramble across a railroad bridge to reach the university campus. The first structures were built atop marshy land crisscrossed by Indian trails and thick with willow, poplar, and scraggly brush. The earliest buildings were broad, plain edifices made of the local yellow sandstone, which spoke of practicality and substantiality. Across the North Saskatchewan River, on a rise by the bank, the ornate provincial legislature building was taking shape.

One of Tory's arguments for the establishment of a medical faculty had been based on the need for doctors in rural areas. When practitioners arrived from the East, they tended to set up practice in the urban areas, leaving the majority of Alberta's population without adequate medical care. Tory suggested that only locally raised physicians would appreciate the needs of the sparsely distributed population and would return to their small communities to practise. In some ways, Collip's students would practise as their predecessors had the century before, treating their patients in their homes and travelling great distances over unpaved roads. In the summer, motor cars might serve, but when winter snows and spring thaws made these roads thick with mud and deadly ruts, practitioners had to resort to the old standbys of travel by horseback and sleigh through sparsely settled brush.[18]

When Collip arrived in Edmonton, he was only twenty-two years old, still boyish looking, and terribly shy in front of his medical students. He returned briefly to Ontario that first December to marry his sweetheart, Ray, who had just completed her bachelor of arts that spring. Some of his students learned of his wedding and wrote "Congratulations Dr Collip" on the blackboard when he arrived back in Edmonton. Collip blushed madly and rubbed the note off the board. One former student recalled that, despite his shyness, Collip was an excellent teacher, full of enthusiasm for his subject and able to talk lucidly for an hour without the use of notes. His early attempts at teaching did not always go smoothly, though. In January of his first year, a number of third-year medical students made an official complaint to Herber Moshier. It seems Collip may not have been quite as reliable as his students wished. They listed their young professor's faults: he did not always start lectures on time, he gave no notice to the class when he was unavailable to lecture, and he did not give work with sufficient regularity.

Therefore, they claimed, they were not entirely to be blamed for the low average standing on their Christmas test. These students were in their final year at Alberta before heading off to the more established medical schools to complete the final years of training. Some were afraid that they might disgrace themselves in front of "the men in Eastern colleges." In his own defence, Collip suggested that he had had to surmount many difficulties in this first year that the class had failed to appreciate. He argued that those who complained had a poor attitude to their work. By way of illustration, he noted that he had set aside the last portion of a course for individual experimentation but had found that only half the class attended regularly and that the other half came in at the end of the period just to inspect the results of the other students. His medical students, with much more pressing and practical matters in mind, seem not to have taken up the ideal of research to the extent he had hoped.[19]

Typical sophomoric fun and even the excitement of encountering new ideas now had to compete with the war in Europe for the students' energy. At university, many students and faculty enlisted for service. Collip's department head, the ever-vigorous Herber Moshier, was given a leave of absence to volunteer for war service in 1916. After his departure, Collip was left carrying all the teaching duties in physiology, biochemistry, and pharmacology. The physical facilities at Alberta were primitive compared to those at Toronto. Because there was no medical building, all the teaching was conducted in the Power House. During this time, Collip's only assistants were practising physicians who served as part-time demonstrators in the laboratories. This left Collip little time for the research he loved so much. His only publication from this period was a review of work on internal secretions that he presented to the Alberta Medical Association in 1916. Consisting of a short resumé of what was known about the function of the endocrine glands, the paper briefly discussed their value for practical medicine. It is one of the few indications that Collip had an interest in hormones and their relation to human health.[20]

SUMMER TRAVELS

One of the problems faced by the faculty members at Alberta was isolation from the larger medical and scientific communities. Travel to the cities of central Canada was expensive and time-consuming. Few guests came west to the "frontier." The university library subscribed to several medical journals, but these were circulated in a slow and cumbersome fashion. As a result, the instructors and students had to develop their own ways to keep abreast of the current literature. Collip was among the founding members of a medical journal reporting club that met to share a meal and present abstracts of recent scientific articles.[21]

Collip also took advantage of opportunities to travel during his summers. These breaks from his routine afforded him interesting and varied experiences and a reprieve from his heavy teaching duties. He was readily inspired and influenced by the ideas and methods of those he encountered, and he could become quite enthusiastic about something new he had picked up. In his early years at Alberta, his research work continued along the same lines it had taken during his graduate studies, but it was also influenced by people he met and the materials available to him. During his summers, Collip travelled to the Research Station of the Biological Board of Canada at Departure Bay, Nanaimo, on Vancouver Island. After his first trying year at Alberta, he spent from late June to early August at Nanaimo collecting specimens of salmon and investigating their pigmentation. The following summer, Collip visited the University of Chicago, partly to use the extensive library facilities. During another summer at Nanaimo, he assisted Newton Harvey in his study of the problem of luminescence, collecting a marine aluminescent worm that came to the surface on a certain day in midsummer each year in order to spawn.[22]

The war was, however, a dark, fearsome backdrop to these events. The University of Alberta had a student body of only 440 when the war started, but by its bloody end, some 484 students, staff, and faculty had gone into active service and 82 had been killed in action. Khaki became common around campus after a Canadian Officers Training Corps was established there. Many students, particularly medical students, were trained through the military medical corps. Herber Moshier, showing the same energy he had in peacetime, organized the 11th Field Ambulance unit to be staffed by students from the four western provincial universities. Students who served in this corps could receive university credit for their service at the front. Moshier, a captain and later lieutenant-colonel, took his unit to the Somme. Just months before the end of the war, he was hit by shrapnel while driving an ambulance and killed instantly.[23] The war hit close to the family as well. Only four months after Reg Turnbull had married Ray's sister Maude, the young divinity student joined up along with his whole class, volunteering to go as a regular soldier rather than as a chaplain. The following year he was killed, lost along with the more than ten thousand Canadian casualties at Vimy Ridge. Maude, widowed so young, never married again.

In 1918 Bert and Ray had their first child, a daughter they named Margaret Mary. Photos show the youthful new father proudly hovering over his baby's pram, his eyes aglow. The new aunts, Ray's sister

Maude and Bert's sister Rita, each made trips out west to visit the latest member of the family. Rita was now a student at Trinity, too. She trained to become a teacher like her mother and, after graduation, taught Greek and Latin to many generations of high school students in Port Credit.[24]

At the close of the war, returning soldiers began to fill the classrooms and strain the medical school's resources. In 1920 the provincial government approved the plans for the construction of a new medical building to house the faculty. That same year, the Rockefeller Foundation awarded $5 million to assist the development of medical education in Canada. The older schools – Toronto, McGill, and Dalhousie – received $1 million each. Alberta, as yet unproven, was granted the interest from an endowment of $500,000. This supported Tory's ambitions to stimulate medical research and scientific and clinical teaching.

With demobilization, Arthur Long came into Collip's life. Long had operated a bookstore in Norfolk, England, before emigrating to Canada. He had farmed for a few years and was a carpenter's helper during the construction of the university. After the university was built, he had been hired as a general laboratory assistant by Moshier. He served during the war as an orderly room sergeant and after 1919 returned to his post in the physiology department. Long was to became Collip's loyal factotum for many decades, keeping the laboratory in order and the morale of its inhabitants high.[25]

The end of the war also brought expanded opportunities for travel. Collip spent the summer of 1919 in Britain visiting Professor Noël Paton at Glasgow and working in the laboratory of Professor J.B. Leathes at Sheffield. Leathes was then conducting a study of the effect of sleep and awakening on carbon dioxide tension of air in the alveoli of the lungs and the rate of excretion of acid and basic phosphates by the kidney. Collip served as a guinea pig in this study, sleeping at Leathes's home so that he could be awakened at given intervals and have specimens of his alveolar air taken immediately.

Collip found his experiences in Britain extremely stimulating, and he began a flurry of investigations of his own that led to the publication of seventeen papers the following year. He was so impressed by the type of experimental procedure that Leathes employed that when he returned to Edmonton, he proceeded to use his own students as experimental subjects in a similar study. He examined the effect of prolonged hyperpnoea (abnormally deep or rapid breathing) on the rate of excretion of phosphates and ammonia and on the concentration of carbon dioxide in the blood. Some of the students entered into the spirit of things so vigorously that they went into muscle spasms of tetany. In his experiment, Collip used the recently published van Slyke apparatus for determining the carbon dioxide content of bodily fluids. With his student Percy Backus, he extended his study to the alkali reserve of blood plasma and to other bodily fluids in dogs.[26]

During the same period, Collip also prepared four articles on the problem of osmotic pressure between blood cells and their fluid medium. This line of research bore the imprint of Macallum's influence: the study was concerned with surface tension phenomena and the transport of solutes across membranes and it employed microchemical techniques. Later that year, Collip undertook a number of studies of the action of adrenalin. This may have been stimulated by his interest in trying to locate adrenalin in nerve cells while doing his master's thesis research. In this work, he prepared extracts of many mammalian tissues – heart, lung, spleen, liver, brain, cord, pancreas, skeletal muscle, testes, small intestine, pituitary, thymus, thyroid, and parathyroid – and tested their ability to make uterine and intestinal muscle contract.[27]

The next summer, he again visited the marine biological station at Departure Bay, Nanaimo. There, he extended his study of the carbon dioxide concentration in bodily fluids to the marine forms he took from the vicinity of the station. His shooting, fishing, and clam-digging trips provided him with a great variety of research subjects – medusae, sea anemones, starfish, sea urchins, barnacles, clams, lampreys, fish, and snakes. He made a special study of anaerobic respiration in the edible clam.[28]

This period of active research was marred by an unhappy development in the department. Since his arrival, Collip had been steadily promoted, first to assistant professor in 1917 and then to associate professor in 1919. Having held down the department on his own throughout the war, Collip felt himself the obvious candidate to take over the headship of the department. When in 1920 Tory decided to hire Ardrey W. Downs from McGill to replace Moshier, Collip viewed this as a grave personal insult. (A colleague ventured the suggestion that perhaps Tory considered Collip too young and inexperienced to take on this position, though in fact Collip was the same age – twenty-seven – that Moshier had been when he died.) This was not the first clash of this sort at the medical faculty. The year before, Tory had incurred the ire of Daniel Revell, the first member of the faculty and the professor of anatomy, when he appointed Allan Rankin to the deanship. Rankin had only been professor of bacteriology at Alberta for a few months before he went overseas for war service. Revell, like Collip and most of the others of the small group that held the school together during the war, was a Toronto graduate. Rankin and most of the postwar appointments were McGill graduates, as was Tory. Revell suspected that old school loyalties might have influenced Tory's decision.

Collip was particularly aggrieved by Downs's appointment because he felt that it reflected upon his own teaching and research abilities. To make things worse, he thought of Downs as ten years behind the times in his research. The incident was to cause friction between Tory and Collip for some time. Collip's bitterness was so intense that on Downs's first day at Alberta, Collip exchanged angry words with him.[29]

In October 1920 Tory requested a Rockefeller Foundation Travelling Fellowship for Collip. Perhaps this was to make up for Collip's hurt feelings in the hiring of Downs[30] or to serve as a reward for bearing the responsibility for the whole department during the war. Certainly it was to give him exposure to new ideas and techniques. One month later Collip learned that he had won the fellowship. What he could not know was that this fellowship would transform his life.

The Discovery of Insulin, 1921–1922

Usually, the first really significant discovery gives direction to the whole subsequent life of its discoverer.

Hans Selye, *From Dream to Discovery*[1]

The Rockefeller Travelling Fellowship gave Collip a chance to set aside his teaching duties for fifteen months. During this time, he would visit and study with distinguished scientists and devote himself to the research he loved so much. When the award was announced in November 1920, Collip began to make his plans. He considered travelling to work with men such as Sir Henry Dale and William Bayliss in London, Benjamin Moore in Oxford, Donald van Slyke at the Rockefeller Institute in New York, Yandell Henderson of Yale, and J.J.R. Macleod in Toronto. He hoped to spend this time learning more about the chemistry of respiration and the chemistry and physiology of the glands of internal secretion. After some reflection, he settled on spending his first six months with Macleod in Toronto, then six months with van Slyke in New York, and finally four months with Dale in Hampstead.[2]

Collip was at an early stage of his career, but he was already demonstrating a great deal of ambition and tenacity in his negotiations with his administrative heads. He was one of a new generation of scientists, trained in original investigation and fully expecting to make research a significant part of his academic career. University of Alberta president H.M. Tory was in some ways very sympathetic to Collip's goals but found it was not always easy to provide conditions suitable for research. Tory was a true institution builder and a scientist himself. Although he had long been away from the physics laboratory, he was a strong proponent of developing the laboratory sciences, particularly if they could be linked to utilitarian purposes.[3] In the Faculty of Medicine, the teaching of medical students remained the staple function.

Despite the Rockefeller benefaction to the faculty, funds for extra staff, equipment, and conference travel were scarce. Collip put up a long struggle over many years to eke out more time and resources for his research work.

By the autumn of 1920, Ray was expecting their second child, and Bert grew more concerned about providing for their growing family. After some bargaining with Tory, he negotiated a sabbatical leave from Alberta with very generous terms. In addition to his Rockefeller fellowship, he would receive a $1,000 bonus to augment the stipend to the level of his full salary. In addition, he secured Tory's promise that he would be promoted to full professor on his return and made chair of a new department of biochemistry that was to be split off from physiology. Tory's final words to Collip before he left on his Rockefeller fellowship were to chastise him for his "propensity to negotiate for financial considerations." Tory warned him not to "say or do anything that can possibly be construed as self-seeking" in his dealings with the Rockefeller officials, since Collip would be risking aid to other people besides himself. Collip assured him that he would exercise discretion.[4]

In April 1921 Collip returned to Toronto to study with J.J.R. Macleod, professor of physiology and a renowned authority on carbohydrate metabolism. His wife and two young daughters travelled with him – Margaret, their first child, and their baby, Barbara, born that winter. Once installed at Toronto, Collip settled into the study of the effect of pH on the concentration of sugar in the blood.[5] His old mentor, A.B. Macallum, was no longer at Toronto; he had become the first full-time chairman of the Honorary Advisory Council for Scientific and Industrial Research, a body created in 1916 in support of the war effort. This group soon became the National Research Council of Canada.

While the ostensible reason for Collip's sabbatical leave was to broaden his research experiences, he also used the time to cultivate new contacts and career opportunities. In May he wrote back to Alberta to his dean, Allan C. Rankin, informing him that he had received three excellent job offers since leaving Edmonton. Only a month into his fellowship, it appears Collip was already considering staying on in Toronto rather than returning to Alberta. He told Rankin that he had received an offer of a "real post" as associate research professor of physiology under Macleod. The plan had only fallen through at the last minute because of a cut in the research spending of the provincial government. Macleod had advised him to instead take the position of assistant professor of pathological chemistry under Victor J. Harding. Collip and his Toronto colleagues had agreed that he should certainly remain for the next teaching year. The question of whether or not he would stay longer was left open. This change in plans required Collip to alter the terms of his fellowship. He decided to spend the summer of 1921 at the Marine Biological Laboratory at Wood's Hole on Cape Cod and at the Rockefeller Institute for Medical Research in New York City. He would then take the entire school term at Toronto and spend the final summer of his leave with Dale in Britain.

Collip used the offer by Toronto as leverage with Alberta. He assured Rankin that he had not given up his intention of returning to Alberta, but, he intimated, "It is true I have been advised by different men not to go back under any consideration as a much bigger future is presenting itself in the East. However I know Alberta a little better and also its possible future also my heart is in the school there." He warned, "Obviously however, if the University wishes me to return it will have to be on a slightly different basis than the one suggested before I left." He described the very satisfactory situation he was promised at Toronto: he would have eight hours of work per week, the help of two demonstrators, and all sorts of facilities for research, including dogs, a fully equipped operating room, chemicals, and glassware.[6] Since Tory was travelling in the East, Collip asked to meet with him in Macleod's office to discuss the Toronto offer.

BANTING'S IDEA

Another visitor to Macleod's lab that May was a young surgeon, Frederick Grant Banting. Banting, almost exactly a year older than Collip, had served as a medical officer in France and Britain during the last years of the war and then, upon his return, had set up a practice in London, Ontario. Since business had been slow in his new practice, he had taken a part-time job as a demonstrator at the University of Western Ontario. Banting had been preparing notes for a talk on carbohydrate metabolism when he came across research on diabetes mellitus. The author of this research study, American pathologist Moses Barron, suggested that the cause of diabetes, as many other researchers were beginning to believe, could be traced to the cells of the pancreas known as the "islets of Langerhans." The pancreas has two types of cells: acinar cells and islet cells. Acinar cells secrete digestive enzymes into the intestines and are thus considered an external secretion of the pancreas, since the gastrointestinal tract is considered (oddly, on the face of it) external to the body. Scattered amidst the acinar cells, like tiny islands, are the so-called islet cells, whose function was still unclear at the time of Barron's study. Could it be that these cells produce an internal secretion, that is, a substance that is released into the bloodstream? And could the activity of this internal secretion have something to do with whether or not someone became diabetic? A number of researchers began to think so. Since the late nineteenth century, physiologists had been exploring the internal secretions of the glands, secretions such as thyroxin from the thyroid and adrenalin from the adrenal glands. These internal secretions, or "hormones" as physiologist Ernest Starling named them in 1902, were defined as chemical messengers capable of setting off physiological responses in organs far from the location in which they were produced.

In the case study that Barron described, a stone had blocked the pancreatic duct so that the acinar cells had atrophied. Interestingly, the islet cells had remained intact. Banting reasoned that if the islets of Langerhans were somehow related to diabetes, he should find a way to separate their activity from the digestive function of the surrounding acini tissue. Perhaps if one were to tie off the pancreatic duct, one could make the acinar cells die off, as happened with Barron's subject. In his diary entry of 31 October 1920, Banting wrote: "Diabetus [*sic*]. Ligate pancreatic ducts of dog. Keep dogs alive till acini degenerate leaving Islets. Try to isolate the internal secretion of these to relieve glycosurea."[7]

Over the next weeks, Banting was so excited by this idea that he began to pursue it with various colleagues.[8] Since the facilities for a research project of this sort didn't exist at Western, Banting was directed to J.J.R. Macleod, the respected expert on carbohydrate metabolism at Toronto. Toronto was one place Banting might find the resources he would need for such extensive animal experiments. Macleod was initially sceptical about Banting's abilities, finding that the young doctor had only a superficial understanding of the literature on diabetes and little familiarity with the methods of physiological research. After all, this problem was already being studied by a number of skilled researchers in several countries. Many had attempted to isolate the internal secretion of the pancreas before and had failed in their efforts. At length, Macleod agreed to provide Banting with the facilities to test his ideas the following summer. Macleod reckoned that even if Banting could only come up with negative results, these would still be valuable as a contribution to physiological knowledge.[9]

Banting arrived at Macleod's lab at about the same time that Collip came to Toronto. Macleod and Banting seem to have met several times to determine the best course of action Banting could take. Macleod likely suggested that Banting should first familiarize himself with diabetes by removing the pancreas of one or two dogs. He probably advised Banting to try to make acinar cells atrophy by ligating the pancreatic ducts of other dogs. Once Banting had done these things, he could begin to use the internal secretion from these partially atrophied pancreases to treat the dogs he had surgically made diabetic. To test the results, Banting would need to use chemical tests of the blood and urine. Unfortunately, he had little knowledge of these sorts of techniques and would probably require some advice and assistance. Around this time, Banting and Collip first met in Macleod's office. Banting copied Collip's summer address into his notebook, perhaps thinking the biochemist might be someone he could contact should he have any questions about these chemical concepts and procedures.[10]

Since Collip found he was getting some good work done, he remained in Toronto until 16 June, when Macleod sailed off on his vacation. Collip also began his summer travels, first to Montreal, then to New York, New Haven, and Boston. Ray, not deterred by having young children, was his constant companion on these trips. According to Collip's associate Robert Noble, Collip had early on perfected an autoclaved baby formula that allowed he and Ray to tote baby supplies for over a week.[11] Happily, the seaside locations of some of the research stations made them particularly good holiday spots for the family.

Collip spent part of the summer at the marine biological laboratory at Wood's Hole, where he continued his studies on anaerobic respiration in mollusca. He was delighted to be able to gather much data for this study. The atmosphere at the laboratory was highly stimulating, and he was able to discuss his work with such leading biologists as Jacques Loeb, A.P. Mathews, and Ralph Lillie. One of the things he picked up was a new method of blood sugar determination; this he learned from the investigators at the next bench, a Professor Bradley of Wisconsin and his student Elmer Severinghaus, who were studying dogfish. The Shaffer-Hartman technique of blood sugar determination had just been published, and Collip found it so superior to any he had used before that he subsequently refused to use any other method. After Wood's Hole, he travelled on to the St Andrew's Marine Biological Station in New Brunswick to continue his study of anaerobic respiration in the local marine forms. By the end of the summer, he counted himself to have had a very profitable time. He was pleased to be asked to write an article for *Endocrinology*, the official organ for the Society for the Study of the Internal Secretions. He had published some of his physiological studies of adrenalin and one solid review of internal secretions in the *Canadian Medical Association Journal* a few years before. Since he felt *Endocrinology* was a clinical journal (it wasn't entirely, though perhaps it was more so than the physiological and biochemical journals in which he generally published), he considered the invitation a tangible recognition of his published work.[12]

Although his research work flourished over the summer, his private negotiations with Alberta stalled. Collip had arranged a meeting with

Tory in Toronto, but the occasion had been strained. A flurry of letters between the two men followed, full of ugly recriminations. Tory was angry that Collip had changed his travel plans without consulting him. Collip tried to argue that he had only made these changes to get the most out of his leave. He maintained that his spending the winter in Toronto did not mean he was making any commitment to that university. Collip offered, "While as I see it I have an assured future in the East if I care to stay yet I have never changed my opinion of the West."

Tory had asked that Collip keep an eye out for a good candidate to fill a post in the new biochemistry department. Collip was able to report that he had found, not one, but two very good choices, and he suggested that he needed them both. Each of them had a very different type of training, he argued, and he felt that with these two he could build up a real research department, one that could undertake questions not only of academic but also economic importance. Here, Collip was appealing directly to what historian Marianne Ainley calls Tory's entrepreneurial ideology of science.[13] Collip maintained that money alone would not take him back to Edmonton; rather he needed the promise of full-time staff that would allow him to carry out research.

He also wrangled with Tory over the promised bonus of $1,000. By choosing to take the post at Toronto for the year, Collip had sacrificed his stipend from the Rockefeller Foundation for twelve months. He argued that he should keep his bonus, since his decision to stay in the East was not of his own seeking, "but the opportunity offered I embraced it because by so doing I was to spend the year to the best advantage." Collip reminded Tory that he had been "cut to the quick" when he did not receive the headship of the physiology and biochemistry department. After a year of reflection, he claimed that he could now better understand Tory's decision, recognizing that it had only been based on the information available to Tory at that time. Collip submitted that the recognition he was now receiving in the East was beginning to heal that wound.[14]

Unfortunately for Collip, this letter only served to enrage Tory further. Tory chastised Collip for remaining at Toronto and "dropping back into the old groove," as he saw it, after Tory had gone to such effort to win him the opportunity for broader experience. Furthermore, Tory bristled at Collip's continued attempts to bargain for a better position. Tory's appointment of Ardrey Downs the year before – and Collip's harsh and unconcealed opinion of Downs's abilities – continued to be a sore point between Tory and Collip. Tory was shocked by the hostile comments Collip made about Downs during their meeting. Although he was certain these remarks had to be based on a very wrong impression of Downs, Tory was sufficiently upset about them that he had turned to his McGill cronies, men whose judgment he trusted, to be assured that there was no foundation for what Collip had said. He admonished Collip: "That you could repeat about a colleague what you did to me on mere rumour is somewhat startling." Tory explained that although Collip had promptly complained to Tory about what Downs had said to him upon his arrival, Downs had remained silent about Collip's conduct until he was asked directly by Tory. Reproaching Collip, Tory wrote: "The only reason that I refer to these matters now is that it brings into my mind a doubt whether in spite of the many good qualities of mind you possess, you can ever overcome that disposition of seeing matters only in the light of your own desires, a disposition which is recognized by all your old friends."

Tory made it clear that he did not feel that the university owed Collip anything more than it had already given him. He noted that Collip was the only member of staff to receive an eighteen-month leave on full salary. "None of these points seem to have had any effect upon you when you made arrangements cancelling all that I had done." Since Collip was receiving a larger salary at Toronto than the one he had from Alberta, Tory thought the Board of Governors might consider giving Collip a portion of the originally proposed $1,000 bonus but only for the three or four summer months, after he had completed his year at Toronto and before he resumed his position at Alberta. As for Collip's hopes of establishing a research department, Tory strongly reined in his ambitions, making no definite promises: "If I have one ambition greater than another it is that in the next ten years we will build up all the scientific departments into research departments and as far as my strength of mind and body will enable me to get the men and money I will do it." He indicated that he fully wished to provide opportunities for any staff members capable of research but had no intention of singling out Collip's department for special treatment. He concluded, "If you come back to us I want you to come back not in a spirit of bickering but with an ambition to co-operate with your other colleagues in promoting not only your own department but the well-being of the whole University."[15]

Collip, hurt and chastened by Tory's harsh remarks, began to regret his whole conduct since Moshier's death. He wrote back to Tory: "That my loyalty to the University of Alberta for example should for one moment be called into question and all my work and activities be attributed to selfish motives makes me feel pretty sick." He explained in his own defence: "I have often mentioned financial matters to you but I would hate to think that you feel I am a money grabber. I long ago set myself to keep up to date in my work and that can only be accomplished by travel combined with work. I have never spent a summer in my own laboratory yet and my bank account tells the tale.

However, I do feel that I have not lost anything but indeed have gained a great deal by thus getting about."[16]

Tory replied in December with a final offer. Collip was to receive a salary higher than the one he had in Toronto and with a bonus of $100 per month for the following summer, that is, for the final months of his leave after he had departed Toronto. Tory also agreed to put one full-time staff member in the department but left the question of additional assistance for further discussion. Collip would be responsible for four hours of lectures and six hours of laboratory teaching a week, which Tory argued was perfectly reasonable.[17]

When Collip returned to the pathology department at Toronto in the autumn of 1921, he looked in on the work of Banting and Banting's young associate, Charles Best, a recent graduate of the same honours physiology and biochemistry program from which Collip had graduated. Banting and Best had had a very exciting summer while Macleod and Collip had been away. They had been able to produce interesting results by injecting an alcoholic extract of the pancreas into depancreatized dogs. This extract had the remarkable effect of lowering the blood sugar in diabetic dogs. Banting was very pleased with his results and believed that they might be applied to the treatment of diabetes in humans.

Collip found this work promising and on several occasions indicated that he would like to help. Banting thought this a good idea and asked Macleod if Collip might join the research team. During the first months of Banting's project, Macleod had been reluctant to add more hands, but now he began to reconsider, particularly because Banting and Best had made another important discovery. They found that to make the special extract, they did not have to use the labour-intensive method they had devised earlier; that is, they did not have to painstakingly tie off the pancreatic ducts of dogs, wait for the acinar cells (the cells making the digestive secretion) to wither, and then remove the pancreases. Instead, they could simply use the whole pancreases of cattle. Although this meant that the idea that had originally inspired Banting had led up a blind alley, it also meant that they could produce much larger amounts of extract than before thanks to the ready availability of bovine pancreases from the slaughterhouse. Banting and Best had also begun using the Shaffer-Hartman technique of blood sugar determination, possibly at Collip's suggestion. In December 1921, Macleod finally agreed to allow Collip to join the work.[18]

Collip eagerly launched himself into both the biochemical and physiological aspects of the question. His first misstep was to ask the young worker at the abattoir for sweetbreads instead of pancreases (sweetbreads can mean the thymus as well as the pancreas). After this embarrassing problem was sorted out, he progressed very quickly, beginning by following up on Macleod's suggestion that the extract of pancreas be tried on rabbits, particularly those that were depancreatized. Collip soon determined that the extract lowered the blood sugar not only of depancreatized rabbits but also of normal rabbits. This discovery meant that the group now had a quick and easy way of testing the activity of a batch of extract, simply by injecting normal rabbits. After consulting with Banting, Best, and Macleod, Collip then tested whether injections of the extract had an effect on the formation of glycogen in the liver and the excretion of ketone bodies in the urine. Diabetes interferes with the usual metabolism of glucose and fatty acids. Glucose is normally converted to a storage form – glycogen – that is stored in the liver. In diabetics, this important process does not occur and, moreover, fatty acids are only partially metabolized, leaving an intermediate form – ketone bodies – to accumulate in the urine. If the pancreatic extract could be shown to restore the function of converting glucose to glycogen and to eliminate ketone bodies in the urine, this would be an additional indication that the extract served to replace the factor missing in diabetics.

On 21 December, a few short weeks after starting the work, Collip observed that when he injected a depancreatized dog with the extract, its urine was free of ketone bodies. When he dissected the dog, he found that its liver was full of glycogen. These experiments were very significant. They took the experimental proof of the extract's potency beyond the blood and urine sugar readings that Banting and Best had depended upon up to this point. Changes in blood sugar might easily be attributed to other causes, such as the toxicity of the extract. Collip's experiments demonstrated clearly that the extract actually acted on the key metabolic functions that were missing in the diabetic.[19]

During the Christmas break, Banting, Best, Macleod, and Collip travelled down to New Haven, Connecticut, to report their findings at the meeting of the American Physiological Society. There, Banting gave his and Best's first public presentation on the subject. The response of the attending scientists seems to have been one of cautious interest; they had some serious questions that the Toronto group would have to answer if they were to make their results fully convincing. Unpolished, awkward, and inexperienced, Banting had a difficult time defending his work in front of the audience of physiological experts. At a crucial moment, Macleod stepped in to respond to the questions and to rescue the presentation. This only humiliated and angered Banting, sparking his suspicion that Macleod was trying to take credit for the work of the group.[20]

Collip, on the other hand, was very hopeful about his own research and working vigorously. In January 1922, he conveyed his tremendous excitement in a letter to Tory. And, perhaps betting that his research success might be an additional bargaining chip, he again sued for better terms. He thanked the president for his latest offer and admitted that he had been on the verge of accepting it when he had, on that same day, been offered the chair of biochemistry at Dalhousie and, later, a research post at Toronto, sweetened with $500 from a special Rockefeller fund. He suggested that since the University of Alberta had a similar Rockefeller fund, his salary might be topped off with a similar contribution. He argued that given geography and his plans to attend some important international meetings the following year, any Alberta salary was worth $500 less than the same amount from Toronto. On a more positive note, Collip recounted the results of his research, which vindicated – he believed – his decision to stay with Macleod:

I will never regret having decided to spend a year near Professor Macleod ... The crucial experiment was tried out just before the Xmas break and the results were so striking that even the most sceptical I think would be convinced. I have never had such an absolutely satisfactory experience before namely going in a logical way from point to point into an unexplored field building absolutely solid structure all the way. However to make a long story short we have obtained from the pancreas of animals a mysterious something which when injected into totally diabetic dogs completely removes all the cardinal symptoms of the disease. Just at the moment it is my problem to isolate in a form suitable for human administration the principle which has such wondrous powers the existence of which many have suspected but no one has hitherto proved. If the substance works on the human it will be a great boon to Medicine but even if it does not work out a milestone has at least been added to the field of carbohydrate metabolism ...

To be associated in an intimate way with the solution of a problem which for years has resisted all efforts was something I had never anticipated. I only wish that the various papers which will be published on this work were coming from Alberta rather than Toronto. A whole new field has been thrown open however and I will continue to work along these lines for some time no doubt.[21]

He closed on a conciliatory note, heartily thanking Tory for the concessions made to him by the board: "I have been in the West long enough to have imbibed the Western spirit. I am desirous of returning to it even though it may not present all the immediate advantages offered in the East."[22]

Tory replied, congratulating Collip on being associated with such a weighty problem, especially one connected with human health. This was precisely what he, Tory, had wished when he had contacted the Rockefeller people. As for the terms of Collip's post, though, no better offer could be made.[23]

In the meantime, the research work had been progressing at a rapid rate. Banting was beginning to feel pushed aside by the professional researchers, Macleod and Collip. In his anxiety, he persuaded Macleod and Duncan Graham, Eaton Professor of Medicine at the university and head of medicine at the Toronto General Hospital, to allow a clinical trial of the extract that he and Best had made. The test of 11 January proved a failure. The extract had only a small effect on the blood sugar of the patient, and because it contained impurities, it caused a sterile abscess at the point of injection. This premature clinical trial became yet another source of friction among the members of the group. Although they had all pooled their results previously, Banting was turning his and Best's work on purification into a competition with Collip's work.[24]

Around this date, Collip made another very significant discovery. He had observed that a large dose of the extract sometimes caused his rabbits to go into convulsions. The wretched animals would shake violently, then collapse, only to have seizures again and again every fifteen minutes until they finally died. When Collip first encountered these convulsions, his initial assumption was that the extract must be toxic in some way. Observing a convulsing rabbit one day, he suddenly had another idea. He quickly drew a sample of blood and set it aside; then he grabbed some glucose, mixed it with water and injected the animal with the solution. The rabbit recovered. When Collip later analysed the hastily drawn blood sample, he confirmed what he had suspected: there had been almost no sugar in the rabbit's bloodstream. He had discovered the phenomenon that would later be called insulin shock. The extra-large dose of extract had caused the body to empty too much of the sugar from the blood. Collip's glucose injection had countered this by raising the blood sugar to a more normal level. This story comes from O.H. Gaebler, who witnessed the events. He commented: "It all looks simple now, but it was the most thinking per square meter per minute that I have seen."[25] After that dramatic demonstration, Collip was always very careful to warn clinicians of the potential danger of insulin overdose.

Amidst all the excitement in the laboratory, Collip had to deal with some grave problems at home. The new baby, Barbara, went from illness to illness. First, she had rickets, then diphtheria, and by winter, she had come down with pneumonia. At one point, Collip worried that she might die. Then, Ray and both daughters succumbed to the flu. To avoid getting sick himself, Bert enlisted his sister-in-law, Maude, to serve as nurse to his young family while he camped out in the lab on a cot. Alas, poor Maude came down with the flu herself while caring for the Collips.[26]

Collip was thus conveniently set up to work both night and day. He continued with his most important task of purifying the extract for clinical use. On 19 January he found himself once again alone in the laboratory, still working on the problem. He had been experimenting with various solvents in an attempt to separate the active principle from contaminants in the crude extract. On this night, he fiddled with different concentrations of alcohol. He found that he could get most of the contaminants to drop out of solution by increasing the concentration of the alcohol. Finally, he increased the alcohol solution to a concentration of 90 per cent. Suddenly, the elusive active principle precipitated out in pure form. Beside himself with excitement, Collip ran up and down the empty corridors. He telephoned Ray to tell her that he "had it."[27]

Collip's success, as marvellous as it was for the project, sparked a confrontation with his co-workers sometime during the next few days. Although there are no contemporary accounts of what happened, historian Michael Bliss was able to piece together some of the story from versions recorded by Banting and Best decades later. It appears that Banting was threatened by the thought that his work was being taken away from him just as it was coming to fruition. Collip, perhaps wary of Banting's distrustful attitude, announced that he had discovered how to purify the principle and that he did not intend to share his secret with Banting and Best. He might even take out a patent on it. Banting, already insecure, was pushed beyond his limits. The two men had an angry confrontation and almost came to blows. Clark Noble, a student and research assistant to Macleod, drew a cartoon, now lost, entitled "The Discovery of Insulin." It showed Banting sitting on top of Collip, choking him. Shortly after, on 23 January, a clinical test was made of Collip's extract. This time, the results were clearly positive.[28]

For those of us at the beginning of the twenty-first century, a time when diabetes is generally thought of as a chronic but not fatal condition, it is perhaps difficult to fully appreciate the drama of this achievement. Until 1922, a diagnosis of diabetes mellitus was a death sentence. Young children stricken with the disease could expect to live only a few years. Their bodies, unable to utilize the carbohydrates they ingested, would gradually waste away. The glucose passed through the body unused, making the patient urinate frequently and be consumed by a fierce thirst and hunger. The excess sugars in the blood would slowly poison the body, sometimes resulting in blindness, foot and leg infections, and even gangrene. The best treatment that diabetologists had been able to develop was a stringent low-calorie, low-carbohydrate diet. Patients able to adhere to these diets might be able to buy a few months, even a few more years of life, but would slowly, steadily starve to death if they did not die of diabetes. In the spring of 1922, the Toronto group and their clinical collaborators began to test insulin on more and more patients. Some sufferers came to them almost living skeletons. The lucky ones who received insulin in time responded by gradually regaining weight, strength, and vitality. Clinical photographs show a stark contrast between the diabetic children before treatment, emaciated and listless, and their robust, even chubby selves, full of life, only months later, all because of insulin. Michael Bliss calls it "the closest approach to the resurrection of the body that our secular society can achieve."[29]

A few days after the clinical trial of his extract, Collip wrote to Tory telling him that he would be pleased to accept the terms that Tory had set out. He related the news of the "phenomenal break" in his research: "The problem seemed almost hopeless so you can imagine my delight when about midnight one day last week I discovered a way to get the active principle free from all the 'muck' with which it appeared to be inseparably bound." Since the clinical trial had proved so encouraging, $5,000 was immediately put at the disposal of the team to secure apparatus and four assistants to rush the work and try to build a block of clinical evidence. On the advice of Macleod and others, Collip kept the process a secret until it was fully tested. If the material proved satisfactory, he would direct the planning of the manufacturing process with the university's Connaught Laboratories.[30]

BRINGING INSULIN TO THE WORLD

It was now clear that the discovery was of immense importance. Macleod turned over the resources of his department to the project, and on 25 January the group signed a formal agreement to work collaboratively with the Connaught Anti-Toxin Laboratories. The Connaught labs had been set up in 1914 to produce vaccines and antitoxins for public health use. Banting, Best, Macleod, and Collip agreed that none of them would attempt to patent the product independently. The step of formally setting down the principles of cooperation was probably precipitated by the angry and confusing confrontation between Best and Collip of that week. Their antagonism had underlined the need to spell out the technical and financial details of the collaborative work.[31] Collip dropped the rest of his sabbatical plans and devoted himself to the problem of the large-scale manufacture of the extract, now officially named "insulin."

After the initial excitement was over, the mood in the laboratory turned bleak for several months. Biologically active extracts are notoriously finicky to make, and soon after his great triumph, Collip discovered that he could no longer make the potent extract. It is difficult to determine why there was a problem. Variations in vacuum pressure, temperature, and distilling time can all wreak havoc on a temperamental extract. Also, Collip's casual way of note taking may not have helped. He tended to jot down the details of his extraction recipes in a little black notebook that he kept in his back pocket.

Eventually, he, Banting, and Best recovered the ability to make insulin, but they were also forced to recognize the limitations of their operation. The work at the Connaught Laboratories had been fraught with difficulties. By May the news of their work had drawn the attention of many in the medical world, and Banting and Macleod were now deluged with heart-breaking appeals for supplies of insulin. Production at the Connaught could not keep up with the growing demand. The group decided to accept the invitation of the pharmaceutical firm Eli Lilly & Company to collaborate in the work. Lilly could offer the research staff, facilities, and funds that the Toronto group would not have access to otherwise. Lilly's research director, George Clowes, was himself a research chemist and had been very interested in the Toronto group's work from the time he had heard Banting deliver his paper at New Haven.

The question of whether a physician should profit from the sale of a medical product caused considerable debate during this period. Macleod and Banting were concerned about contravening medical ethics by patenting their discovery, but they also recognized that if they did not do so, they risked losing control of insulin to a competitor. In April the group decided to apply for a patent in the names of Collip and Best and then assign the patent to the university. The next month, the group hammered out an agreement with Lilly that gave the company the rights to manufacture and sell insulin in the United States and Central and South America. The firm was given an exclusive licence for a period of one year, during which information on any improvements was to be pooled between the Toronto group and Lilly. Large-scale clinical trials would be made in Toronto and the United States, and Lilly would provide the extract for these tests free of charge at first and later at cost. In Britain and the rest of the empire, the patent rights were to be offered to the British Medical Research Council. The university Board of Governors set up a committee – later to be called the Insulin Committee – to deal with managing the patent and licensing process. The patent application had initially been made in the names of Collip and Best because they were the two non-medical members of the group. Later, Banting was persuaded to add his name as well because the patent was at risk of being voided on the grounds that Collip and Best were not the sole inventors. The American patent was issued on 23 January 1923, and the Canadian and British patents were also awarded.[32]

At the end of May 1922, the members of the group read papers at the meeting of the Royal Society of Canada.[33] The insulin team then broke up, as Collip's appointment at Toronto was ending. In early June, Best and Collip travelled down to the Eli Lilly headquarters in Indianapolis to share their knowledge of producing insulin with the Lilly staff and to help with the first attempts at extraction.

Collip returned to Edmonton shortly afterward to take on his new position as the chair of the Department of Biochemistry. He had been privileged to participate in what was the most important achievement in Canadian medical research. Collip's contribution had been vital to the success of the Toronto group. Banting and Best admitted that before Collip's arrival, their results had been no better than those of previous investigators. In finding a way to purify insulin and then to demonstrate its physiological activity, Collip had taken their work beyond what had been achieved by the several other researchers who had tackled the problem before. Collip had made several important contributions to the understanding of insulin's physiological effects: he developed an assay for insulin in normal rabbits; he identified the hypoglycaemic reaction; and he showed that insulin helped restore the body's ability to store glycogen and to eliminate ketosis. Michael Bliss argues that "without Collip's work insulin might well have been isolated somewhere else."[34] While the interactions of the four principal participants in the insulin work had been bitter and fractious at times, it was nevertheless their collaboration that had led to their success. Now, only a few months short of his thirtieth birthday, Collip returned to Alberta, his career transformed. The discovery of insulin had become the event that would define the rest of his professional life.

3

The Parathyroid Hormone Controversy, 1923–1927: A Question of Priority

This is the one big thing in my life and it means everything to me to be given credit for my discovery. You will realize, I am sure, that I consider it no trifling matter when I am wrapped up in it heart and soul ... It is far more than a question of money. It is immortality.

Adolph M. Hanson to Harvey Cushing, 15 April 1925[1]

Collip's career had taken a dramatic turn with the discovery of insulin. From that point on, he would be assured a place in the research world, but now he had to capitalize on the advantages he had gained. Over the next years, he worked assiduously to create another triumph like insulin, his research program turning decisively towards the extraction and characterization of hormones of therapeutic value. In his pursuit of this goal, he demonstrated the many lessons he had learned from his Toronto experience.

When Collip returned to the University of Alberta in the summer of 1922, he knew that his circumstances were greatly changed from those he had left the year before. In Toronto the insulin discovery was gaining wide public attention and attracting many diabetics to the city. Although Banting had found himself somewhat on the sidelines during the later development of insulin in the laboratory, he now established a central place for himself in the clinical use of the hormone. Banting was the figure that patients and their doctors would associate with this new treatment, and his supporters in the medical community were successful in ensuring that, to the world, the names "Banting and Best" were synonymous with the insulin discovery.

Despite this, Collip gained recognition from his peers in medical science as well as from his fellow western Canadians, who regarded him as a local hero. To westerners, it was regional bias that led to the neglect of their man by the Toronto medical establishment and the "eastern" press.[2] Collip was applauded by medical groups and celebrated in local papers. He was honoured at a special banquet in Edmonton and at a luncheon in Calgary. The University of Alberta awarded him its highest degree, a doctorate of science.

Then, in October 1923, the Nobel Prize was awarded to Banting and Macleod. This was the first time the prize had been given to North Americans. Banting, whose enmity with Macleod had intensified, was furious that he had to share the award with Macleod and that his loyal friend Charlie Best had been neglected. Banting immediately made the public gesture of sharing half his prize with Best. In a dramatic move, Macleod followed suit by announcing that he would share his prize with Collip to indicate that Collip's contribution had been equal to that of the others.[3]

Although Collip was personally hurt by the quarrels that had marred the triumph of the discovery, and although he failed to receive as much credit for his contribution as Banting and Best had for theirs, his association with the achievement proved to be a tremendous boost to his career. Donations and grants poured in. These funds allowed him to follow up on his insulin work and to hire a research assistant. The College of Physicians and Surgeons of Alberta donated $9,000 to his research efforts; the Rockefeller Foundation awarded him $5,000; and the Carnegie Foundation gave $10,000. More significantly, Collip, like Banting, Best, and the University of Toronto, had a share of the insulin royalties. Over the next decades, an era before large-scale government funding was available, these royalties would prove to be a substantial and relatively reliable source of research funds for the three discoverers. As early as 1925, Collip's portion of the royalties amounted to $8,000.[4]

NEXT STEPS

At the Alberta medical faculty, important steps were being taken to upgrade scientific and clinical teaching. The medical course was expanded to a six-year, full degree–granting program. In 1922, just nine years after it had opened, the school received a class A rating from the American Medical Association (AMA) Council on Medical Education and Hospitals. That same year, the urgently needed new medical building was completed. Upon his return to Edmonton, Collip was able to move out of the old Power House and into his new quarters there. The biochemistry department was located on the west half of the third floor, while anatomy was on the east half.

Collip found his new laboratory space a great improvement over the makeshift accommodations he had had before. He had even gained a spacious animal room that was well lit, heated, and ventilated. Soon, however, his expanding research program was stretching even these facilities to the limit. The animal room was scarcely sufficient for the several hundred dogs he went through in a year, let alone for all the rabbits and other small animals. By 1926 the crowded conditions and somewhat disorganized laboratory management were causing problems. A dog tethered to a desk wreaked havoc in the laboratory. Sinks were allowed to get dirty and overflow, flooding the laboratory a floor below. Solving these problems called for some quick improvisation. Collip even considered using the lecture room next to his office to house his small animals.[5]

Collip's first interest upon returning to Alberta was to manufacture insulin for clinical use and to oversee continued experiments on it. Confident of the importance of his work, he made it clear to President Tory that he expected Alberta to match the good facilities he had enjoyed at Toronto: "As the problem I am now working on is such a big one and of such practical importance I will be only able to give it proper attention if I have adequate assistance."[6] He soon began work on an insulin-like substance that he extracted from plants. This substance – "Glucokinin," as he called it – looked tremendously promising as an alternative source of insulin.

Tory was dedicated to fostering research in all university departments in an equitable manner, but he now had to accept that the work of his most illustrious faculty member would have to receive special attention. He reported to the Rockefeller Foundation in 1923: "As you know Dr. Collip is continuing his work in connection with Insulin and Glucokinin and we are getting for him from special sources the money that is required to make his work all it ought to be."[7] For example, unlike the members of other departments, Collip received a lot of assistance. In the meantime, there was very little extra funding for anyone else. Ralph Shaner was an anatomist from the Harvard Medical School who, according to Elise Corbet's history of the university's medical faculty, worked "quietly and diligently" for many years and gained an international reputation in cardiac embryology. In sharp contrast to Collip, he had little financial support and had to make do with small grants of $150 in 1932 from the Banting Research Foundation and $75 in 1935 from the Carnegie Corporation.[8]

Collip continued to benefit from his association with his mentor, A.B. Macallum. Macallum served as the first chairman of the National Research Council in 1917 and then took up the chair of biochemistry at McGill University in 1920. He supported Collip's nomination to a Fellowship in the Royal Society of Canada as early as 1922, but in 1925 Collip still had not been elected. When Macallum noted that Collip's name was left off the list of nominees (by mistake, it was later discovered), he was furious. He threatened to ask his own son,

A. Bruce Macallum, to withdraw his name from nomination because he felt it was unjust that the younger Macallum be considered when Collip was not.[9]

In 1924 Sir Arthur Currie, principal of McGill University, wrote to Collip in confidence to ask if he would consider joining the Department of Biochemistry as "second" under A.B. Macallum. Currie promised that Collip would assume the chair after Macallum's retirement. He suggested, "I know you are head of the Department at Edmonton, but yet I feel you would not regard joining a department presided over by Macallum, who is the doyen of Bio-chemists, as something which your prestige would not allow you to do."[10] Collip declined the invitation, explaining that he preferred to live in a smaller city now that he had a young family. His third child, a son John, was born in 1924. Moreover, he continued, "to be perfectly frank I wish to remain at Alberta for some little time yet. I have spent a number of years now in building up a department and it is only now that I have a satisfactory organization. I would therefore like to be enabled to reap the benefits of this." He outlined his terms: "I take it that the post which you suggest is a teaching post in his department. I have already gone through quite a mill of teaching and am now enjoying what is practically a research post since I have sufficient staff to handle most of the arduous work of teaching. If at a later date a research post should become available at McGill and you should then care to consider me I would be very glad to consider an offer."[11]

The discovery of insulin had been a turning point in Collip's career. Having had a taste of research that so directly and dramatically saved human lives, he found he could not return to his more abstract studies of leeches and clams. He moved away from general physiology and bio-chemistry – from the investigation of fundamental processes in a wide range of organisms – and devoted his attention to the investigation of hormones, particularly those of value in medical therapeutics. As a sign of this new orientation, he enrolled as a medical student at Alberta. This no doubt created a somewhat awkward situation for his instructors, since he was a fellow faculty member and department head. Of course, Collip was not required to take the basic science courses, but he had to complete the final two years of the six-year program. He received his MD in 1926, but he had to graduate one year after the rest of his class because he hadn't assisted in enough deliveries to pass his course in obstetrics and gynaecology.[12]

In his subsequent investigations, Collip followed the pattern established in the insulin work. In the laboratory, he honed the skills that he had used so effectively in the chemical extraction of the hormone and in the physiological assay of its effects. His insulin experience had also taught him the value of patenting the products he developed and of collaborating with pharmaceutical firms. When he discovered new principles, he sought arrangements for their production similar to those that the insulin group had made with Eli Lilly.

GLUKOKININ

Collip's first venture was to find a source of insulin other than slaughterhouse animals. He was not alone in this search. Macleod, Clark Noble, and N.A. McCormick investigated the teleost fish as a source. Best and D.A. Scott looked into plant tissues. These researches caused some concern at Eli Lilly, and its scientists began to investigate many alternate sources of insulin as well.[13] Collip returned to an organism with which he was already familiar – the clam *Mya arenaria*. He postulated that since insulin served to convert glucose to glycogen, a hormone similar to insulin would be present wherever glycogen appeared in nature. The clam was one lower animal that was rich in glycogen. In December 1922 Collip returned to Toronto to attend the meeting of the American Society of Biological Chemists and the American Physiological Society. There, he and his insulin colleagues presented papers on their insulin work. Collip also presented his first paper on this insulin-like substance. He reported that he had used the same method of extraction on clam tissue as he had used in insulin extraction and had produced a preparation that caused a normal rabbit to go into convulsions upon injection. As with insulin, these convulsions were relieved by the injection of sugar. When he used a modified version of the extraction method, the blood sugar did not fall until several days after the administration of the extract, and sometimes only after an actual rise in blood sugar.[14]

Collip speculated that there might be similarities between the plant and animal kingdom, and he turned to a more readily available organism – yeast. On 26 January 1923, after many months of failure, he finally succeeded in preparing a yeast extract that produced marked hypoglycaemia in normal rabbits. When he injected a depancreatized dog with the extract, its blood sugar fell to a normal level and its urine was sugar-free. Encouraged by this success, he extended the work to plants that did not contain glycogen or starch; he was soon busily extracting everything from onion tops, and onion roots to barley roots, sprouted grain, green wheat leaves, bean tops, and lettuce. In March he announced that his new plant hormone was to be called "glucokinin." He stated emphatically, "That this new hormone will be useful in the treatment of diabetes mellitus in the human subject there can be little doubt." In fact, he claimed, this substance would in some ways be much superior to insulin because the effect took more time to develop and lasted longer.[15] That same month, the Cambridge team of L.B. Winter and W. Smith announced that they had independently obtained similar results with yeast extracts. Anxious not to lose credit for this new work, Collip cabled off a note to *Nature* in April explaining the course of his studies and arguing that Winter and Smith shared coincident priority with him.[16]

In Toronto, Macleod was sceptical about the value of these findings. He worried that Collip had foolishly rushed his results into print before working through the other possible interpretations of the results. For example, the hypoglycaemic effect might have been caused by damage to the liver, or the glucokinin might have been stimulating the normal rabbit's own pancreas to produce more insulin. He was particularly annoyed that Collip had so hastily made a claim to priority with Winter and Smith.[17] By April, Collip, too, realized that there were problems with his experiments. The public claims he now made about glucokinin began to sound more provisional. He noted that some of the extracts had been toxic and that when the toxicity problem had been overcome through the use of weaker extracts, the hypoglycaemic effect was less striking. The blood sugar measurements had looked promising, but when he had attempted to measure the glycogen content of the liver, he found that there was none. Furthermore, the extract caused an initial rise in the amount of sugar excreted in the urine, and only after that did the urine become free of sugar. The action of glucokinin proved quite different from that of insulin. With insulin, the fall in blood sugar occurred shortly after injection and reached its low point two to six hours later; glucokinin sometimes took days to take effect. Because of a lack of apparatus and time, Collip was not able to conduct the tests of respiratory quotient and ketone excretion, tests that had been so important in characterizing the effect of insulin. He admitted in a paper, "The author fully realizes that the experiments herein set forth are far from complete as yet and, therefore, not without criticism, but the results so far obtained have been so uniform in character that a preliminary paper on the work done to date seemed justified." As for the clinical use of glucokinin, he reported that extracts of such purity had been produced that an actual test on a diabetic subject was planned, but remarked that the therapeutic value of the hormone remained to be demonstrated.[18]

Collip continued with a long-term experiment that involved keeping a depancreatized dog alive with glucokinin extract as Banting and Best had with insulin. The effects of a single injection seemed to persist for so long that Collip feared that a small piece of pancreas might have been left in the animal and was continuing to regulate the blood sugar.

The animal died at the end of sixty-six days, and a post-mortem examination performed by Daniel Revell, professor of anatomy, seemed to vindicate Collip. Revell could find no trace of pancreas upon gross examination. By June, however, Collip admitted that he "had lost faith in the experiment" and that clinical trials would be postponed until more facts about the physiological response could be determined.[19] In demonstrating that glucokinin had an effect on blood sugar, Collip had progressed only as far as Banting and Best had with insulin before Collip had joined the team. Collip was well aware that blood sugar changes might be induced by all sorts of other substances, including toxic ones.

His final full paper on the subject was submitted in June. In it, he pursued an interesting phenomenon that he had uncovered while working with glucokinin. After an animal developed hypoglycaemia following an injection of glucokinin, he took a blood sample and injected it into a second animal. He observed that the second animal quickly became hypoglycaemic as well. When he separated the blood components, he found that the same effect could be created by transferring the blood serum portion alone. He also found that the principle could be transmitted through a series of animals. Furthermore, this transmission effect occurred even when the initial hypoglycaemia was caused by substances other than glucokinin. The animals experienced the typical symptoms of hypoglycaemia, such as weakness and convulsions, but unlike insulin shock, these symptoms were relieved only for a short time by the administration of glucose and the ultimate result was always death. He named this phenomenon "animal passage hypoglycaemia."[20] After this paper, he remained silent on the subject. For a time, he continued to search for the answer to this strange problem, but eventually he moved on to other subjects. Four years later, he published a note admitting that he had never been able to duplicate his earlier results. He felt it his duty to report that he now believed that the effect must have been caused by an organism transmitted in the serum.[21]

After the disappointment of glucokinin, Collip published very little for almost a year. In the summer of 1924, he again travelled to Nanaimo to study the effect of insulin on the oxygen consumption of marine fish and invertebrates.[22] Otherwise, his research program became devoted almost exclusively to mammalian subjects, in particular the special problems of human physiology and health.

THE PARATHYROID HORMONE

Collip's next venture was the isolation of the parathyroid hormone.[23] This work added a new triumph to his record but also embroiled him in a bitter priority dispute with a Minnesota physician, Adolph Hanson. In many ways, this fight was reminiscent of the insulin turmoil.[24]

During the late nineteenth and early twentieth centuries, the study of the endocrine glands emerged as an experimental science, breaking away, from the practice of organotherapy. Merriley Borell argues that this development was accompanied by a gradual change in methodology.[25] In the organotherapeutic tradition, the internal secretions of the glands were thought of as potential treatments for disease and their presence was indicated by clinical results. In the new science of endocrinology, hormones were conceptualized as chemical messengers and their presence was proven by the production of standard physiological and biochemical changes in experimental animals. Diana Long Hall argues that the tension between these two approaches constituted a major theme in the history of endocrinology and continued to play a role in shaping related intellectual and institutional matters into the 1920s.[26]

Even as the new science was establishing an institutional basis, however, expectations for the therapeutic value of the internal secretions outran scientific understanding. Not only was organotherapy exploited by quacks and charlatans; it was also widely and uncritically applied by enthusiastic physicians in Britain and America. Laboratory scientists strove to distance themselves from this side of endocrinology by emphasizing the physiological bases for these organotherapeutic cures. The discovery of insulin and its use in the treatment of diabetes mellitus brought a new legitimacy to hormone therapy, stimulating large-scale research on the hormones of the other glands. There were already extracts of the hormones adrenalin and thyroxin, but the discovery of insulin had a particularly dramatic impact, offering the first real hormone treatment for a disease that was neither rare nor readily controlled. In the 1920s and 1930s, the isolation of new hormones became the focus of such intense competition that research in this field was likened to a gold rush.[27]

THE RISE OF THE SCIENCE-BASED PHARMACEUTICAL INDUSTRY

The science-based pharmaceutical industry was also becoming an important factor in medical research. By the 1920s some of the larger firms had built sizable research staffs. These firms were beginning to regard scientific research and development as a way of gaining legitimacy and a competitive advantage in the marketplace. Their scientific activities helped to differentiate them from the vendors of quack remedies.[28]

Collaborative ventures between industry and academic scientists could yield benefits for both parties. An academic scientist who discovered a new therapeutic agent and wished to apply it to practice required the assistance of a pharmaceutical firm, since universities seldom had the facilities to manufacture drugs on a large scale. The firms were able to provide the research staff and resources to help in developing the rudimentary product to a form in which it could be industrially produced. The academic scientists and their universities were also able to apply royalties to the support of research. This was particularly important in an era before large-scale government funding of medical research. In return, the pharmaceutical houses could profit greatly from the inventiveness and expertise of the university scientists. The cooperation between the University of Toronto and Eli Lilly & Company in the development of insulin was a celebrated example of successful collaboration.[29]

During this period, greater numbers of medical scientists and pharmaceutical firms began to use the patent system to protect their products. The issue of whether to patent medical products was a new and difficult one for both academic scientists and industry, as the medical ethics of the time demanded that medical products be donated to the common fund of knowledge and not be used for profit. Attitudes of medical scientists towards medical patents began to change. One motivating factor was their desire to protect the public by controlling how the product was to be exploited; another was their wish to keep the profits for further research. The course taken by the Toronto group – handing the insulin patents over to the university – became an increasingly accepted way of accomplishing these goals.[30] The administrators of these patents could exert some measure of control over the price, manufacture, and distribution of the product while adding to the research funds of the university.

COLLIP'S EXTRACT

Before 1924, investigators had demonstrated that when the parathyroid glands were surgically removed, the patient would experience generalized muscle contractions (tetany) and die. In clinical practice, this was of concern because parathyroid glands were sometimes accidentally damaged or removed in thyroid surgery for goitre. The most common treatment for tetany, and an effective one, was calcium salts taken by mouth. Other researchers attempted to treat tetany with extracts or grafts of the parathyroid gland as well. Several commercial preparations of desiccated parathyroid products were also available, although most of them were of dubious value.[31]

The two chief theories concerning the function of the parathyroid glands were (1) that these glands had a role in the regulation of calcium metabolism and (2) that they detoxified methyl-guanidine, a poison that was an end-product of bacterial putrefaction in the intestines. In 1909 William MacCallum and Carl Voegtlin produced evidence in support of the first theory, demonstrating that parathyroid tetany could be corrected by the administration of parathyroid extract or by the injection of calcium.[32] Noël Paton and his colleagues at the University of Glasgow were the principal proponents of the second theory. In 1916 they produced a series of papers demonstrating that the convulsions of animals with parathyroid tetany were similar to those of animals injected with guanidine. The Paton group's conclusions were primarily based on similarities between the animals' convulsions and the clinical symptoms in humans.[33]

In mid-1924, Collip began his investigation of the parathyroid hormone. What made Collip interested in the parathyroids? One of his colleagues recalls that in the summer of 1919 Collip showed a great deal of interest in this area of research after meeting Noël Paton in Glasgow. Collip had also worked with Leathes at Sheffield on the effect of sleep and awakening on the blood chemistry. In the two papers Collip had published on this work, he tied tetany to acid-base balance and calcium deficiency. Winter and Smith, with whom Collip had claimed coincident priority on the yeast insulin-like hormone, published a paper discussing a possible relation between the pancreas and the parathyroids. They observed that parathyroid extract seemed to augment the hypoglycaemic action of insulin.[34]

Collip began his study of the parathyroid gland by undertaking an extensive survey of the parathyroid literature, paying particular attention to the debate over the calcium regulation and guanidine detoxification theories of parathyroid function. Perhaps extrapolating from his successful experience with insulin, he decided in favour of the hypothesis that the parathyroid secreted a hormone that controlled blood calcium concentration. If this hormone existed, he was determined to prepare it for replacement therapy.[35]

Many of Collip's colleagues talked about his having something of an intuitive gift for working with proteins; he seemed able to sense just what solvent was called for or when a shift in the pH was needed. Collip also used sheer volume to optimize his chances of extracting active principles. In his parathyroid studies, Collip worked with batches of seventy-five to one hundred glands at a time.[36]

By October 1924 he had some promising results. Using hot hydrochloric acid, he had made a crude extract that could be used to control tetany in a parathyroidectomized animal. In the following months, he attempted to further purify this product by varying the alcohol and ether concentrations with isoelectric precipitations and filtrations. He also experimented with different methods of administering the extract. This work was complicated and required a great deal of animal experimentation. Collip was fortunate to have the resources to perform dozens of experiments on dogs, but there were problems with many of the animals. Several never developed any sign of tetany after thyroparathyroidectomy and could not be used for the experiment; others died from tetany or infections. Collip nevertheless succeeded in finding examples of complete replacement therapy in which the thyroparathyroidectomized dogs were maintained for many months on parathyroid hormone. Treatment was withdrawn and the animals were subjected to tetany; then they were given the hormone extract and allowed to recover completely. This process was repeated many times.[37]

These tests proved that the extract could be used successfully in replacement therapy. But Collip went further. He provided evidence that the relief of tetany coincided with a rise in the serum calcium level. Furthermore, he tested the effect of the extract on normal animals and discovered that it elevated the level of blood calcium. An administered overdose led to profound hypercalcemia and sometimes death. Collip and his research associate, the chemist E.P. Clark, recognized that it was critically important to be able to measure slight changes in blood calcium levels. One of their most notable achievements, and one of the keys to their success, was the development of an accurate quantitative method to determine serum calcium.[38]

While Collip was primarily concerned with the biochemical and physiological aspects of this work, he was also mindful of the potential therapeutic value of the extract. Only two months after his first recorded animal experiments, he had an opportunity to carry out a clinical trial of his preparation. Collip and D.B. Leitch, a physician on the faculty of the University of Alberta, reported in the *Canadian Medical Association Journal* that they had successfully treated a young child stricken with infantile tetany. They conceded, however, that it was difficult to determine the uses and limitations of the new hormone with such limited clinical data. They also recommended the careful monitoring of blood serum calcium to avoid overdose.[39]

Before he had even published his results, Collip contacted representatives of Eli Lilly & Company. He was of course familiar with the firm, having worked with Lilly in the development of insulin. By early December 1924, Collip submitted his first report to the *Journal of Biological Chemistry*. What he did not know was that a Minnesota physician named Adolph Hanson had developed a method of making parathyroid extract by hot hydrochloric acid as well. In fact, Hanson had taken his product to Lilly several months before. Just before Collip sent off his paper, George Clowes, director of research at Eli Lilly, sent a telegram informing him of Hanson's work and urging him to make some mention of Hanson's findings in his publications.[40] Collip inserted a footnote citing Hanson's papers in *Military Surgeon*. He remarked that "Hanson's attempts to prepare an active extract of the parathyroid glands of animals are worthy of great commendation" and that "his clinical results are indeed highly suggestive."[41]

ADOLPH M. HANSON

Adolph Melanchton Hanson (1888–1959) was a medical practitioner who had been drawn into experimental investigation out of an enthusiasm for science and a concern for his patients. In this respect, he could be thought of as coming from a long and fine tradition. During the 1920s, however, the archetype of the lone physician-scientist was being challenged by the emergence of a new profession, one to which Collip belonged, that of the career scientist associated with research institutes, academic and industrial laboratories. How did someone like Hanson view this new scientific establishment from outside its ranks?

Hanson had received his early training at Hamline University and the University of Minnesota. He had then earned his MD at Northwestern University in 1911. In 1917 he trained at the school of neurosurgery at the University of Pennsylvania and then went overseas with the U.S. Army Medical Corps. He served as a surgeon at Evacuation Hospital No. 8 under Harvey Cushing, one of the leading figures in American neurosurgery and endocrinology. Hanson later published several papers on the neurosurgical techniques that he had developed during the war. Returning home after the war, he settled into private practice in the town of Faribault, Minnesota. In his spare time, he continued to pursue his scientific interests, taking first a bachelor and then a master of arts degree in chemistry with E.O. Ellingson of St Olaf College in the nearby town of Northfield. In 1922 he set up a small laboratory in the basement of his home to carry out his experiments. Hanson's research work was very much a family enterprise. His children recall taking turns at the kitchen meat grinder to help him prepare an extract of the bovine thymus gland that he used to treat cancer. They also remember having to endure many meals made up of the surplus sweetbreads, although they reported that their mother's butter and cream sauces made them somewhat more palatable.[42]

Two years before Collip started his study, Hanson had already begun to work with the parathyroid gland. Hanson's interest in the subject arose from his experience with thyroid operations for goitre, during which the nearby parathyroid glands were sometimes accidentally damaged or removed. Hanson entered into the work hoping to determine the chemical composition of the gland and perhaps isolate an active principle. If he succeeded in finding a new substance, he intended to carry out animal experiments to test it.[43]

Soon after he began his studies, Hanson developed his method of hot hydrochloric acid extraction. He devised the procedure by adapting various standard tests of chemical composition. The extract he produced through this method appeared to contain an organic principle that he named the "Hydrochloric X." In March and April of 1923, he published his first papers describing the chemical composition of the gland and outlining the various extracts he had derived.[44]

As an independent researcher, Hanson had to spend long hours in the slaughterhouse collecting small batches of eight to twelve glands. He did not have the facilities to keep and use experimental animals and was therefore unable to test the physiological effect of these extracts. He struggled to enlist the aid of investigators in academic laboratories, succeeding first with A.W. Bell at the Department of Pathology of the University of North Dakota. Bell enthusiastically reported that the Hydrochloric X relieved the symptoms of tetany in four animals.[45]

In 1924 Hanson presented a paper to the Minnesota Branch of the Society for Experimental Biology and Medicine and published several more reports in *Military Surgeon* detailing his method of preparing the extract and describing Bell's experiments. As his research progressed, Hanson became more and more convinced of the value of his extract. He persuaded other academic researchers, such as Arthur Hirschfelder, head of the Department of Pharmacology, Edward Kendall of the University of Minnesota, and Frederick S. Hammett of the Wistar Institute, to test his extract. Their findings were negative or, at best, "suggestive but in no way conclusive."[46]

While Hanson clearly wanted to make his work scientifically legitimate, he lacked the expertise and resources to overcome many of the obstacles. Furthermore, as a medical practitioner, he felt that the therapeutic value of his work was of greater significance. Influenced by the ideas of H.W.C. Vines, M.D., a Foulerton research student at the Pathological Laboratory of Cambridge University, Hanson began to use his extract on his patients. He embraced Vines's suggestion that parathyroid extract, in addition to being useful for tetany, might be of value in treating such problems as infections, ulcers, and tuberculosis. These were the sorts of ailments Hanson's patients brought to him daily. Full-blown tetany, on the other hand, was relatively rare; he had never seen a case himself. Hanson became more and more convinced of the therapeutic value of his extract, and on 18 June 1924 he contacted

Eli Lilly and urged the company to take up the study of the Hydrochloric X. In November that year, Lilly chemist H.W. Rhodemhamel notified Hanson that he had indeed begun work on purifying the extract.[47]

THE DISPUTE

In Edmonton, Collip began spreading the news of his discovery. He published widely in Canadian, American, and British journals and presented news of his work at many of the key conferences of the medical and scientific professions, such as those of the American Physiological Society, the American Medical Association, the American Congress on Internal Medicine, and the National Academy of Science.

Collip also continued his scientific study of the hormone. By April 1925 he reported that he and his associates had carried out over 250 animal experiments in their efforts to trace the physiological effects of the hormone. In July of the same year, he and Clark published an improved method of purification: the extraction with boiling hydrochloric acid was followed by salting-out with sodium chloride and several isoelectric precipitations. Finally, Collip and Clark challenged the guanidine intoxication theory of parathyroid function. Unlike Paton and his associates, who had used an analogy of clinical symptoms in their argument, Collip and Clark used direct physiological means to test the theory. They compared the nitrogen and urea curves of the blood of parathyroidectomized dogs with those of dogs injected with guanidine and found that the changes in blood chemistry were distinctly different. They argued that this was conclusive proof that parathyroid tetany was not caused by guanidine intoxication.[48]

Collip provided other experimental workers with samples of his extract to allow them to explore its biological activities. He also supplied the extract to many clinicians for clinical trials. Over the following year, he was conservative in his estimation of the therapeutic applications of the hormone, stating that it was known to be effective only in the treatment of hypoparathyroidism, particularly post-operative tetany. Post-operative tetany, while a rare occurrence, could be sufficiently severe that treatment with calcium lactate was ineffective. In these cases, the parathyroid hormone offered new hope. Although Collip had reported in his early papers that the hormone was effective upon oral administration, he later had to retract this claim. In further studies of the chemical properties of the hormone, he discovered that it was rendered physiologically inert by the action of the digestive enzymes, pepsin and trypsin. Collip also continually warned clinicians of the danger of overdose, which he found could lead to death in laboratory animals.[49]

As a result of his efforts, Collip gradually established himself as an authority on the subject. In 1927 he was asked to write an article on the parathyroid hormone for the *Journal of the American Medical Association* in its series on glandular therapy. Collip's paper was followed by an article by William McCann, written to replace the one McCann had published three years earlier. McCann testified that three years before, in 1924, he had not felt that any claims for the therapeutic efficacy of parathyroid preparations could be justified, given the published evidence. These reservations extended to the early work of Hanson. But now, in 1927, McCann could assert with confidence that an effective agent was available. He argued that although Hanson had "described the preparation of extracts of parathyroid of which some must have contained the active principle,"[50] Collip and his co-workers had now provided clear evidence of the method of extraction and the description of the physiological action of a parathyroid hormone. Furthermore, the clinical reports confirmed the value of the Collip extract as a therapeutic agent.[51]

Hanson was livid when he discovered that Collip's method and product were essentially identical with his own.[52] He felt that Collip had not given him proper recognition. He wrote to Harvey Cushing explaining that while he did not want to deny Collip his due, he felt that it was only good sportsmanship that he also be accorded credit for accomplishing the first stage of preparing the hormone. He began to feel that the Eli Lilly firm had not dealt fairly with him, as Lilly's people had known of Hanson's work before they had taken up Collip's product. In anger, Hanson turned to the rival pharmaceutical firm Parke-Davis for help. On 30 March 1925 he made an application for a patent for his product and immediately assigned the patent rights to Parke-Davis. While Hanson found the idea of patenting a medical product distasteful, he felt it was necessary to protect his priority. He wrote passionately of this to Cushing:

This is the one big thing in my life and it means everything to me to be given credit for my discovery. You will realize, I am sure, that I consider it no trifling matter when I am wrapped up in it heart and soul. I carried on this work as an independent investigator and paid for the expenses out of my private purse. I almost ruined my health and worked many times all night, while I was forced to care for my practice on which my livelihood depends. I have no doubt that the Scientific World will give me credit for my discovery, but a favourable decision by the Patent Office will only render this more sure. It is far more than a question of Money. It is immortality.[53]

Hanson began to recognize the limitations of his scientific work. He had depended too much on his clinical findings (for example, that his

extract created a sense of well-being and added strength), and his animal experiments had only demonstrated that the symptoms of tetany
had been relieved. Now, the value of the scientific facilities and staff of
Parke-Davis became clear. To strengthen his case, Hanson worked with
the scientific staff at the firm's laboratory in Detroit. This time, in addition to documenting the relief of symptoms in the animals treated, the
research team carefully measured the serum calcium at regular intervals. Axel Hjort and his associates at the Parke-Davis laboratory confirmed both Hanson's and Collip's results by making detailed tests of
the extraction of the parathyroid by various solvents at different concentrations and temperatures. They also set about preparing a purified
product, carrying out the painstaking work of standardizing it, and ini-
tiating clinical trials.[54]

To Collip, who had so recently been embroiled in the bitter controversy over the credit for the discovery of insulin, this situation must
have seemed painfully familiar. The parallels of the episode to the insulin discovery are striking.[55] In each case, Collip, the professional
research scientist, was caught in a bitter conflict with a small-town
physician who had embarked on research work with less advanced scientific training. Banting's success, like Hanson's, was perhaps due as
much to incredible perseverance as to scientific expertise. Both of Collip's adversaries had reacted fiercely when they perceived that the credit
for their work was being taken from them. More significantly, each of
them had accomplished the first stage of the extraction of the hormone
and had primarily regarded the extract as a therapeutic agent. In both
cases, Collip's role as a biochemist had been to purify the extract further, develop a method of biological assay, and demonstrate the presence of the hormone through an examination of various physiological
responses. These distinctions cannot be drawn too rigidly, however.
Banting, too, had demonstrated the effect of insulin on blood sugar,
and in both the insulin and parathyroid work, Collip had been anxious
to use his product in therapy.

Collip acknowledged Hanson's work in his publications, but in a
manner indicating that he thought Hanson had stumbled across the
right answer but had yet to demonstrate it satisfactorily. He allowed
only that Hanson "undoubtedly must have had some of the active principle in certain of his extracts," since he had used the method of hydrochloric acid hydrolysis.[56]

The Lilly staff began to realize that they had a very delicate situation
on their hands and a very tough opponent in Hanson. Like Parke-
Davis, Lilly had invested a large sum of money in purifying and manufacturing the product, in making contacts with a considerable number
of physicians, and in supplying these physicians with samples of the

product. By April 1925 Lilly scientists had improved on the product and obtained a material purer than the original Collip product by three or four times and purer than the Hanson product by ten times. Clowes admitted to Tory that the Collip and Hanson products were equal in yield and potency; they differed only in that the Collip extract had the advantage of a somewhat lower nitrogen content. If Hanson were to win the patent and assign the rights to Parke-Davis, Lilly could very well lose its investment. The firm would either have to use a process that did not infringe on the patent or give up making the product altogether. As soon as Clowes learned of Hanson's decision to patent, he wired Collip, strongly urging him to recognize Hanson's work "fully and unreservedly."[57] Clowes warned Tory that Hanson was liable to "make an open scandal if Collip fails to recognize his work or attempts to deal with him in any casual manner with the intimation that since he prepared an acid extract it probably contained the active principle, or anything to that effect."[58] Efforts at negotiation between Lilly and Parke-Davis and Hanson had failed. Hanson was so angry, he explained to Hjort, that he felt the time had passed for compromise. He refused to have anything to do with Lilly unless it severed all connections with Collip with regard to the parathyroid extract.[59]

For a time, both firms sold parathyroid extract. The University of Alberta Board of Governors agreed to allow Lilly the exclusive right to manufacture and sell the extract in the United States under the proprietary name "Para-Thor-Mone." The university maintained the right to offset any advantage of monopoly Lilly might gain by fixing the price from time to time through arbitration. Also, all materials were subject to testing under Collip's direction in the university laboratories.[60] Parke-Davis marketed its own product under the trade name "Paroidin."

The private correspondence between Hanson and Parke-Davis staff suggests that the firm's representatives were not averse to fuelling Hanson's sense of outrage against Collip and Eli Lilly. Axel Hjort advised Hanson in his dealings with Lilly, suggesting that he present a paper at an upcoming AMA meeting in order "to let the world know your position in this matter" and perhaps "stem the tide of the Collip propaganda."[61] Hjort also counselled Hanson on how to present himself in his scientific publications. He once wired Hanson to try to prevent him from submitting a paper for publication; he was worried that Hanson would injure his own cause by making broad therapeutic claims based on his clinical findings. Hjort had warned Hanson about this sort of thing before. He explained that the scientific community regarded the claims of researchers like Vines as being the result of irrational enthusiasm and a lack of properly controlled experimentation. Despite this, Hanson again and again lapsed into making claims based on anecdotal clinical observations. Perhaps this was because he was too eager to believe that his product had broader application. In a hopeful letter, Hanson speculated that the parathyroid hormone might be more important a discovery than insulin. Even though Hanson knew that Collip had discovered that the proteolytic enzymes of digestion destroyed the parathyroid hormone, he continued to prescribe the oral administration of the Hydrochloric X as late as 1935. He did so in the belief that his extract contained some useful substance in addition to the hormone. Years later, he continued to report that he found the extract effective against such ills as pulmonary and laryngeal tuberculosis, gastric and duodenal ulcers, wounds, toxemias of pregnancy, arthritis, cystitis, bronchitis, encephalitis, chorea, paralysis agitans, asthma, pleurisy, eczema, hemophilia, nervousness, and even a general feeling of being rundown.[62]

The priority dispute influenced the development of other aspects of the scientific work that occupied the two researchers. Collip and Hanson produced competing methods of biological assay and competing unit sizes for the hormone. Since Lilly and Parke-Davis marketed their products with the unit size chosen by the researcher each of them backed, the scientific literature on parathyroid had a confusion of "Collip Units" and "Hanson Units" for many years. The priority dispute was further complicated by the addition of a third claimant, Louis Berman, an endocrinologist and biochemist from the Laboratory of Biological Chemistry in the School of Medicine of Columbia University, New York. Berman filed a patent for a parathyroid extract on 12 May 1924. His method differed from Collip's and Hanson's, but his early publications did not disclose critical details of his experimental work. After Collip made his announcement the following year, Berman responded by publishing two further reports of his work, more detailed than the previous ones. He challenged Collip's priority in an angry letter to the editor of the *Journal of the American Medical Association* on 23 July 1927.[63]

Meanwhile, Hanson had become even more upset. He verged on accusing Collip of plagiarism, arguing that his own report in the *Proceedings of the Society for Experimental Biology and Medicine* of February 1924 had predated Collip's first recorded experiment by seven months. How valid was Hanson's charge? All but one of Hanson's 1923 and 1924 publications had appeared in the *Military Surgeon*, the journal for the Association of Military Surgeons of the United States; it is unlikely that Collip, an academic biochemist, would have come across them. Hanson's 1924 abstract in the *Proceedings*, however, had been clearly entitled "Experiments with an Active Extract of Parathyroid" and had included a description of the method of preparing the extract as well as a report that it was effective in treating tetany in para-thyroidectomized dogs. Collip was certainly familiar with the *Proceed-ings*, and in fact, after searching the literature in mid-1924, he cited several papers from the journal in his initial publication on the para-thyroid. Notably, he cited Berman's paper on the subject, which ap-peared in an issue of the *Proceedings* following the one in which Hanson's article had appeared.[64]

The historical record offers no conclusive evidence about when Collip first learned about Hanson's method. Written testimonies suggest that it was brought to his attention only in early December 1924, after he had completed his early experiments. Clowes commented to H.M. Tory, pres-ident of the University of Alberta, that he had "wired Collip about Han-son's work early in December [1924] and subsequently wired and wrote him about being sure to at least insert some foot-note regarding Hanson in his earliest publications."[65] Collip added this footnote to his first pub-lication, received by the *Journal of Biological Chemistry* on 3 December 1924: "Since the submission of the data herein recorded for publication, the papers of Dr. Hanson of Fairbault [*sic*], Minnesota, published in the Military Surgeon ... have come to the attention of the writer."[66] Given Collip's skill in extracting the hormones of many other glands and given his laboratory style (described by colleagues as "strangely unorthodox and ... reminiscent of Mrs. Beaton" because "he rarely carried out a pu-rification procedure in exactly the same way"),[67] it seems entirely possi-ble that Collip developed the method of extraction with hot hydrochloric acid quite independently, through a process of trial and error.

Over the next few years, references to the disputed priority were veiled, at least in the scientific literature. In private correspondence, however, Hanson was vitriolic. He began to believe that his enemy was not Collip but "Organized Medicine" as a whole, or rather, the small clique he thought was running the American Medical Association. He felt that this clique readily accepted Collip's claim but refused to recog-nize his own simply because he was a "nobody" from a small town. He speculated that "Organized Medicine" had set up a code of ethics that favoured the career scientist from the world of universities and insti-tutes, foundations and endowments.[68]

Hanson may have been discounted by many professional scientists not so much because he was an independent researcher, but because he was a clinician studying the secretions of the glands. During this pe-riod, the AMA, led by Morris Fishbein, the editor of its journal, was undertaking a crusade against nostrums and medical quackery. One of the chief targets of the campaign was the glandular charlatan. The leaders of the new science of endocrinology were troubled that their work was associated with disreputable glandular treatments. Their problem was compounded by the popularity of organotherapy among practitioners and the public. The recently formed Association for the Study of Internal Secretions, although counting such notable medical scientists as Lewellys F. Barker, Walter B. Cannon, Joseph Aub, Harvey Cushing, and Edward Kendall among its early presidents, experienced considerable scepticism and even hostility from the medical community. Hans Lisser, former president of the association, later recalling the poor attendance at meetings, speculated that endocrinology was in such disrepute that "it might have been safer and wiser to have met in secret." He added, "Conditions were such that any younger clinician, not yet firmly established and despite an unblemished reputation, who dared to embark on a career in this field was looked upon askance, considered naive and gullible or – perhaps worse – suspected of straying into the realm of quackery, and heading for the 'endocrine gold fields.'"[69] Medical scientists were particularly concerned about the well-meaning general practitioner, who was apt to be led astray, they felt, by the bombardment of advertising material. In his presidential address before the association in 1921, Harvey Cushing urged his fellow members to exercise caution: "Endocrinology as a special subject, if it wishes to survive and come to be a factor in medical practice, must look out for the character of its clinical advance agents lest it come to be utterly discredited."[70] In this context of "hazy therapeutics," Collip's discovery was regarded by the editor of the association's journal as "a matter of congratulations," since "it does contain a something that does something."[71]

In the midst of his dispute with Hanson, Collip joined the fight against glandular quackery, if in a modest way. That year, 1925, Collip was elected the president of the Association for the Study of Internal Secretions. Reporting on his address to the AMA, the press carried headlines declaring that the young Canadian scientist pronounced monkey glands to be "buncombe." This was a reference to Collip's comments on the Voronoff glandular treatments. As far as can be ascertained, this was the one public denouncement of quackery that Collip made during his long career. He was perhaps eager at this time to distance his own work on the glands from its less scientific counterpart.[72]

In the scientific literature of the time, Hanson and Collip were sometimes given equal credit for the isolation of the parathyroid hormone, although Collip was acknowledged to have conclusively demonstrated the physiological activity of the hormone through his measurement of the serum calcium. When supporters of either Collip or Hanson referred to the accomplishment, they subtly emphasized the contributions of the man they backed. When scientists from outside Collip's and Hanson's immediate circles used the extract in their research, however, they usually cited only Collip. Over the years, as the details of the episode dimmed with time, references to Hanson's contribution became less frequent.[73]

THE OUTCOME

In a sense, both Hanson and Collip might be considered to have won this dispute, since two distinct battles were fought with two sets of rules for winning. The notions of discovery were construed very differently in patent law than in science. In the outcome of the dispute, the two notions became entangled just as biomedical science and commerce themselves became more enmeshed.

On 21 November 1927, Hanson's patent application was declared in interference with applications from Berman and Collip, and with one other, from a Joseph A. Morell.[74] Berman and Hanson were the contenders with the earliest claims to priority, so the applications of Collip and Morrell were dismissed. At the final hearing on 5 March 1931, Hanson's case was presented by Parke-Davis lawyers and Berman's by Lilly lawyers. Berman's attorneys argued that Berman had priority in this matter because one of the aspects of the invention was the demonstration of the physiological action of the extract on the blood serum calcium; it was doubtful that Hanson knew that his extract had an effect on the serum calcium before Berman's filing date of 12 May 1924. The examiner of interferences ruled, however, that this was merely an incidental property. In awarding priority to Hanson, the examiner explained that it was "not essential to the invention that the inventor should know the reason why the composition accomplishes its purpose or that he should be aware of the particular chemical, physical or physiological properties of the substance which enable it to accomplish that purpose." It was only necessary that the invention be put to useful application, and indeed Hanson had done so, prior to Berman's filing date, by showing that his extract treated tetany. It did not matter that he did not have a clear idea that his principle was a hormone; nor did it matter that he had been unaware that it acted to raise the serum calcium level.[75]

The next battle that Hanson had to fight was to prove that his claim was patentable. Patent law required that an application be filed within two years of the first public disclosure of the invention. The law examiner ruled that Hanson had revealed his discovery in his first publication of March 1923 and that his patent application of 30 March 1925 was therefore invalid. Hanson applied to the Board of Appeals and was in the ironic position of trying to prove that although he had described boiling the glands in dilute hydrochloric acid in this first paper, this procedure had been merely part of the test for purine bodies; he had not known at that time, nor did he have proof, that the method was the same as that for the preparation of the parathyroid hormone. Hanson's appeal was rejected, but his attorneys later had several interviews with the examiner and, according to them, they "finally convinced him that he was in error and that a patent should issue."[76]

On 13 December 1932 the U.S. Patent Office awarded Hanson the patent for the product and process of extracting the principle of the parathyroid gland. Parke-Davis, Eli Lilly, and later E.R. Squibb produced the product under his patent for some years. Hanson finally felt vindicated. Referring to his dual accomplishments of developing the method of extraction and refining and standardizing the product, he penned this colourful analogy: "It seems that I am about to receive the credit for being the first to reach the North and the South poles of the Parathyroid problem (as Amundsen did with the earth and his dogs). Others reached them too, but he was the first one there. He was a crude explorer, but he got there, and he got there first."[77]

As a result of his patent win, Hanson received much attention in the press and several awards from local medical groups. The Minnesota State Medical Association presented him with a gold medal in 1933. He was asked to provide an article on the subject of the parathyroid glands to the *Journal of the American Medical Association*. Sadly, though, he became aware that the scientific community continued to associate the name of Collip with the parathyroid discovery. He was highly sensitive to rumours that others in the medical profession were criticizing him for profiting from a medical discovery. As an independent researcher, he did not have the option available to academic scientists of donating his patent to his university and having the proceeds channelled back into his research. For several years, he had looked forward to using his royalties to finance further investigations. Now, despite the fact that he had drawn his family into serious debt because of his devotion to his science, he felt compelled to donate his royalties to the Smithsonian Institution. Disheartened but still determined, Hanson continued to run the Hanson Research Laboratory for many years, describing himself as patron, chief chemist, assistant chemist, stenographer, bottle washer, and janitor. He worked in collaboration with Parke-Davis in attempting to extract the active principles of many other glands, including the pineal, carotid body, parotid glands, lymph gland, and spleen. The most successful of his later ventures was an extract of the thymus, called "Karkinolysin," which he used in the treatment of cancer and which he found also promoted growth.[78]

Collip can be said to have won the dispute with Hanson in another sense as well. In today's scientific literature, he is the one credited with preparing an active extract, providing conclusive proof of its activity, and opening the field for further research. His modification of the Kramer-Tisdall method of calcium determination and his development of a biological assay are also noted as important achievements. Late in his career, Collip was recognized for the major contributions he had made to the physiology of the field. As a special guest at the first symposium devoted entirely to the parathyroids, he was lauded as a founder of parathyroid research. In 1959 a bronze tablet was erected in the Department of Biochemistry of the University of Alberta in tribute to the international recognition Collip had achieved for his isolation of the parathyroid hormone there in 1925.[79]

Paul Munson, an endocrinologist writing about the priority dispute decades later, suggests that Collip's work was more readily accepted than Hanson's by the scientific community because, to some extent, the growing profession of endocrinology preferred to acknowledge the contributions of a biochemistry professor, with a grand discovery already to his credit, over those of a small-town practitioner and amateur chemist.[80] Certainly, Munson and others are correct in saying that Hanson's case was not helped by his having "buried" his early publications in *Military Surgeon*, where those involved in endocrine research were unlikely to discover them. Furthermore, the credibility of Hanson's claim may have been damaged by the fact that his first report on the preparation of the extract was accompanied by the description of several clinical cases in which he had used the Hydrochloric X to treat a variety of ulcers and infections. More significantly, however, the scientific community's criteria for identifying a discovery could not be met by the simple preparation of an extract; the discoverer had to understand what the extract contained and give scientific proof of its action. To the scientific world, it was not sufficient to just reach the North and South Poles, as it were; one had to actually realize that one had gotten there and had to be able to prove it. Moreover, as endocrinology emerged as an experimental science, the proper sort of proof became defined as the production of standard physiological responses rather than as individual clinical results.

The two pharmaceutical houses that played a part in this dispute were caught between the two notions of discovery. For the purposes of patent law and the commercial exploitation of a product, the demonstration of clinical results was crucial. For scientific credibility, however, the experimental definition was more important. The pharmaceutical firms that wanted to establish reputations as scientifically sound manufacturers of hormone products had to work within the rules of the new experimental science of endocrinology. Using standardized physiological indicators helped these firms differentiate themselves from the producers of desiccated glandular therapies. It also allowed them to manufacture products of greater purity and standardized activity.

After 1932, Eli Lilly & Company agreed to recognize Hanson's rights under the contract with Parke-Davis and proceeded to manufacture and market the product under the Hanson patent. Lilly abandoned its trade name "Para-Thor-Mone" in favour of the "Parathyroid Extract – Lilly," while Squibb marketed it as "Parathyroid Hormone – Squibb." Parke-Davis continued to list the product under the trade name "Paroidin." All three products were described as "Parathyroid Extract – Hanson." Regrettably, the value of the extract was limited because patients frequently became immune to it after repeated doses. Because of this, the competitors dropped out of the market over the years and Lilly eventually became the sole firm to produce the hormone in the United States.[81]

THE LABORATORY, THE CLINIC, AND THE PHARMACEUTICAL INDUSTRY

The interactions among the laboratory, the clinic, and the pharmaceutical industry were important in shaping the development of endocrine research in America in the 1920s. They influenced what scientific data was to be considered significant, who would be able to collect it, how the results were to be expressed, and how these results could be commercially exploited. The relations of the three parties continued to intensify in the succeeding decades.

To the endocrine scientist of the 1930s, the surging popular and scientific interest in the hormones brought both danger and opportunity. Leaders in the young field such as Collip clearly feared that their work would be dismissed by orthodox medical science because it was too closely associated with the extravagant claims and fraudulent commercial products that often attended organotherapy. Their key to scientific legitimacy was to firmly entrench the new research program of endocrinology. The goal of their research was no longer to extract cures for deficiency diseases but to study hormones as chemical messengers that functioned in normal physiology. Accompanying this research program was the new criterion that the presence of a hormone be demonstrated not only by the satisfaction of the requirements of replacement therapy, but by the production of standard, measurable physiological responses. Endocrine therapy presented such potential that many general practitioners were drawn to using glandular products and to conducting their own investigations. The medical scientists feared that the new science might be mired down by such physicians, who, although sincere in their desire to help their patients, might be insufficiently critical about glandular therapies. By changing the criterion for establishing the presence of a hormone from a clinical to a physiological measure, the academic scientists moved the locus of authority from the sickbed to the laboratory. By setting a standard for physiological testing that would demand significant amounts of time, training, special equipment, and experimental animals, they also favoured the scientifically trained, institutionally affiliated, full-time scientist over the independent researcher.

The leaders in the new field had the opportunity not only to add to the scientific understanding of physiological function, but to discover therapies for a whole new range of ailments. As in other fields of medical science, endocrine researchers began to work with the science-based pharmaceutical industry to bring the results of the laboratory to practical application. Collaborative ventures were valuable to academic researchers because they could bring the resources of industrial laboratories to the task of purifying and standardizing hormone preparations. Moreover, royalties from successful products could mean new funds for research. With this new partnership, however, came new difficulties. The technicalities of patent law and the demands of commerce reshaped the manner in which scientific findings were transmitted and the priority for discoveries was established.

4

Rebuilding Medicine at McGill, 1928–1933

I am getting more thrilled all the time about the change, and I only hope that luck in research will continue to follow me. If we can get a research staff together, however, if luck deserts in one place for a time, it may hit in another.

J.B. Collip to C.F. Martin, dean of the Faculty of Medicine, McGill University, 9 December 1927[1]

In 1928 Collip accepted a call to succeed A.B. Macallum in the chair of biochemistry at McGill University. Collip's appointment was part of an overall plan by McGill's administrators to rebuild the reputation of its medical school. For Collip, the move to Montreal ushered in a period of unprecedented activity. His next successful endeavour was one of the first fruits of McGill's ambitious scheme.

At McGill, Collip turned his attention to the complex and rapidly expanding field of the sex hormones. This was a highly competitive arena worldwide, one in which theoretical issues and questions of priority were hotly debated. The tension between science and commerce that he had experienced in the parathyroid hormone episode was even more pronounced in this endeavour. Collip was more than an explorer in the intellectual domain; he was also an entrepreneur negotiating the vagaries of commercial collaboration and private patronage. The commodity he offered was the scientific knowledge he produced, its potential therapeutic applications, and, to some extent, the prestige of medical science itself.

As early as 1924, McGill had sought Collip as a replacement for his mentor, A.B. Macallum, in the chair of biochemistry. Sir Arthur Currie, principal of McGill, wrote Collip asking if he would consider joining the staff with the understanding that Macallum, though "still full of vigor, enthusiasm and usefulness," would resign in a few years and Collip would then be given charge of the department. Currie added, "I believe we are beginning a period of great advancement," citing the opening of the new biological laboratories and the Pathological

Institute, which, he noted, "is generally regarded as the finest Pathological building on the continent, while the Biological laboratories are
concidered [sic] very fine indeed." He added that the school hoped to
announce the establishment of a university clinic and that "in the near
future interesting announcements will be made regarding the departments of Public Health and Psychiatry. I believe that our Medical
School has taken on anew [sic] lease of life and will rapidly regain any
prestige which some critics think it has lost." Collip refused the offer,
replying that he preferred to remain in Alberta for a little time yet to
enjoy the research department he had forged. While he had the highest
respect for Macallum, he did not relish taking up a teaching post under
him and was only willing to go to McGill if he could be assured a research position.[2]

The call came again in 1927. The dean of medicine, C.F. Martin,
wrote to Collip privately in August to again explore Collip's interest,
saying, "I and most of my colleagues would view with favor & indeed
with enthusiasm the possibility of your succeeding to the chair." During this same period, however, Collip was in the midst of negotiations
with the Mayo Clinic in Rochester, Minnesota. Collip had considerable
personal connections with the world-famous clinic, having taken his
daughter there to have her tonsils removed and, more significantly,
taken his wife, Ray, there that year for extensive surgery and a lengthy
stay. The clinic had founded the concept of cooperative private group
practice, and its work was undergoing rapid expansion during this period, having grown beyond surgical work to encompass general medicine and laboratory research. In 1915 the Mayo Clinic had established
a graduate medical school at the University of Minnesota. On 11 August 1927, the clinic's Board of Governors voted unanimously to offer
Collip a position on the staff as professor of biochemistry, in conjunction with the University of Minnesota. The offer had excellent terms: a
proposed salary of $10,000 a year, with a bonus of $5,000 for moving
expenses; an assistant at $3,500 a year; a laboratory technician; a labo-
ratory specially arranged for him; and the understanding that Collip
was to be "an independent investigator" and could run his own laboratory. Leonard Rowntree (who incidentally was a collaborator of
Adolph Hanson's on the parathyroid hormone work) wrote that he
and the staff were all greatly interested in Collip's coming because his
field of investigation was very promising, especially with respect to
clinical applications. He assured Collip that while he would be independent, Mayo researchers were looking forward to working with him
as a team as well. At the last minute, however, Collip turned the offer
down. Although he had already arranged for a house and car in Minnesota, he changed his mind, having come to believe that despite offi-

cial statements to the contrary, he would be expected to work on whatever he was told. That possibility was unacceptable to him.[3]

Collip decided instead to take up the post at McGill. He tendered his resignation at Alberta on 30 August 1927, expressing his deep regret to President Tory and adding that he was not leaving through any feeling of dissatisfaction, "for it is hard to conceive of any place where more kindly consideration could have been afforded one." He noted to Martin at McGill that his considerable travelling expenses, subscriptions to journals, and society dues had all been met at Alberta, "in fact they have been so good to me here that it seems an imposition to leave. In this respect, I must say that Dr. Tory has been perfectly splendid and put not the least obstacle in my path." The position at McGill offered a salary of $7,000 and was to begin 1 June 1928. Currie wrote, "I, personally, am very gratified that the hopes we have had in mind for the last few years have at last been fulfilled."[4]

A.B. Macallum had apparently been delaying retirement for some time. He had encountered difficulties in arranging for a pension because he had been at McGill only since 1920. As well, there had been some difficulty in finding a suitable successor. Macallum had approached I.M Rabinowitch, pathological chemist at the Montreal General Hospital and a pioneer in Canadian clinical chemistry, but Rabinowitch had declined the offer. The position of "number 2" in the department then went to Sidney Bliss of Harvard, but this did not work out well, according to Rabinowitch's recollection many years later. With Collip's appointment, Bliss agreed to remain in the department as long as he could be assured time for research. He continued there for several years. Once Collip agreed to take the job, Macallum felt satisfied that a fine successor had at last been found. He told Collip he was very desirous of being free of the load he had carried for years and was looking forward to having time for his own research; this he intended to carry on "to the very end."[5]

Collip looked forward to taking up his new post with keen anticipation. Only after his appointment was made final did Collip reveal to Martin that he would be bringing with him a considerable research fund. He explained that he had kept silent on the matter because he had not wanted to unduly influence the decision of the McGill administration. Collip's insulin royalties went with him to McGill, and in 1927 they amounted to $13,648. This sum was $2,500 more than the royalties from the previous year; Collip noted that "if it keeps on increasing at this rate, research should not suffer from want of money."[6]

Collip also brought along with him Arthur Long, his "right hand man" since 1915, except during the latter's war service overseas. Although Long owned his own home in Edmonton and, according to

Collip, had been "supremely happy" with his life there, he agreed to follow Collip to McGill as his personal assistant out of sheer loyalty. At McGill, he would play an important role, looking after Collip and facilitating the success of his laboratory group.[7]

Collip's appointment as chair of McGill's Department of Biochemistry was part of a larger plan by McGill administrators to rebuild the prestige of the medical school on the foundation of scientific medicine. McGill's medical faculty was known for the work of Sir William Osler, the great clinician and teacher, but since his departure at the end of the previous century, it had lost ground to the University of Toronto because of Toronto's greater strength in the basic sciences. Toronto medicine had close ties to biology and was influenced by the strong research program that had developed at the university. In contrast, medicine at McGill rested on its strong clinical tradition; furthermore, the instructors in natural history – botany and zoology – did not develop as strong a research-oriented approach to their subject as their counterparts at Toronto.[8] The main elements of McGill's ambitious plan to strengthen scientific medicine in the 1920s and 1930s were the construction of modern laboratory facilities and the appointment of highly promising scientific researchers.

Beginning in the 1920s, the Rockefeller Foundation made a series of grants to McGill, as it did to the universities of Toronto, Dalhousie, Montreal, Manitoba, and Alberta. Marianne Stevens describes how these grants had the effect of catalyzing and reinforcing the reform of Canadian medical education around the science-based model. McGill, unlike the University of Toronto, received almost no financial aid from the provincial government and instead had had to rely primarily on student fees and private support from Montreal's anglophone elite.[9] The grants from the Rockefeller Foundation had a dramatic impact at McGill not only because of the value of the grants themselves, but also because the gifts were made contingent upon the university obtaining additional funds from other sources.

The foundation made significant contributions to McGill's expansion over the next two decades. Grants included a general endowment of $1 million to the Faculty of Medicine in 1921 for the erection of new buildings for physiology, pathology, and psychiatry; an endowment of $500,000 in 1924 for a university medical clinic; $85,000 for research and experimental surgery in 1929; and $1,232,652 in 1932 for development of teaching and research in neurology. This funding made possible the construction of the Biological Building in 1922, the Pathological Building in 1924–25, the Department of Medicine, the University Medical Clinic, and, most notably, the Neurological Institute, which would showcase the talents of the renowned neurologist and neurosurgeon Wilder Penfield. Penfield had been lured to McGill in 1927 with the promise of new research and clinical facilities for his work. The institute, built in 1932, brought international attention and prestige to McGill.[10]

The construction of the new Biological Building in 1922 was an important first step in rebuilding medicine at McGill on the foundation of experimental research. Set on the site of the old medical building, which had been destroyed by fire in 1907, the new five-storey building was constructed with modern laboratory facilities. When the building was opened, four internationally known scientists gave inaugural addresses: Harvey Cushing, Mosely Professor of Surgery at Harvard; Sir Charles Sherrington, Regius Professor of Physiology at Oxford; H.J. Hamburger, Professor of Physiology from the University of Gröningen; and John M. Coulter, Professor of Botany at the University of Chicago. In his speech, Harvey Cushing remarked that with the completion of the new laboratory, "the last word in laboratories had been said," and its creation marked the beginning of the laboratory era in the teaching of medicine. "It is true that similar things are going on in other medical schools, but here at McGill at least, this was the beginning of the laboratory movement whereby the anatomical dissecting room, for generations the only place where observation was called for and the special senses were trained, had come to be largely supplanted."[11]

At the helm of this ambitious rebuilding plan was Charles F. Martin, the dean of medicine and renowned as "a genius for organization." Wilder Penfield remembered him as "a small, quick-moving man who was not at all impressive at first – not until you talked with him and discovered the keen mind, the quick perceptions, the unyielding strength and the human kindness, always served up with a quip or a laugh." He was professor of medicine and a physician at the Royal Victoria Hospital in 1906 and became dean of medicine in 1922. His colleague, D. Sclater Lewis, recalled that by 1930 Martin's reorganization of the faculty was almost complete. In addition to the appointment of Collip in Biochemistry and of Wilder Penfield and his associate William Cone in Neurology and Neurosurgery, Martin had also been responsible for bringing in such renowned medical scientists and teachers as Boris Babkin as research professor of physiology in 1928; R.L. Stehle as head of the Department of Pharmacology; and Jonathan Meakins as the first full-time professor of medicine and director of the new University Medical Clinic at the Royal Victoria Hospital in 1924. According to Lewis, Meakins "breathed new life" into the research work of the clinic. Lewis recalled that "Martin's success as an organiser at McGill had depended on two factors: first, he was a good judge of men and second, he had been able to obtain the funds to attract them to the university. As a result of his efforts, McGill grew less dependent on the Osler tradition and became a first-class medical school in its own right."[12]

A strong supporter of Martin's in his work was McGill's president, Sir Arthur Currie, the military hero who had commanded the Canadian Corps in the last years of the First World War with great success. At the end of the war, he was offered the presidency of McGill University. Although not an academic, he took an active role in the running of the university, from eating with with fraternity men and attending sporting events to personally interviewing all candidates for appointments. In a period before there were vice-principals, assistants to the principal, or public relations officers, his secretary recalls that "the Principal himself really did administer; in his hands were the reins guiding the whole team." Currie was one of the country's leading figures in the postwar years, and his influence and fame proved invaluable to the university's nationwide campaign to raise money to refurbish the facilities that had fallen into neglect during the war. By 1930, however, the Great Depression was beginning to take its toll on the university, and Currie and the Board of Governors had to struggle even to maintain its programs. Nevertheless, Currie actively promoted the expansion of the Faculty of Medicine, most notably by personally supporting its bid to win the Rockefeller gift to build the Neurological Institute in 1932. He did not originate or guide specific plans, but many at the medical school appreciated his contributions of energy and enthusiasm.[13]

By the end of 1928, Martin was able to report that his plans for the medical faculty were going well and that his new staff was settling in happily. As acting principle during Currie's absence, Martin wrote Currie that "everything ... in the Biol. Bldg. is booming & is *most* encouraging. Collip & his staff, Babkin, Stehle etc. all enthusiastic & happy." Babkin was lecturing to enthusiastic groups of students, and Penfield was "captivating everybody and his surgical work on the nervous system is simply marvellous." Martin was only concerned that Penfield was working so hard that "he is going to rapidly kill himself if he doesn't cut down in some way or other." He added cryptically that "Collip and Babkin are measuring up well, as we expected, but the former is certainly temperamental and needs occasionally the benefit of a child guidance clinic."[14] Is this perhaps an indication that Collip's tendency to self-promotion was incurring some ire at McGill as it had at Alberta?

Collip's research work flourished in this new environment. During the period of transition from Edmonton to Montreal, he had produced a small number of papers on a variety of topics, none of which had developed into anything of particular promise, but now he forged into the rapidly expanding field of the sex hormones.

One of the keys to Collip's success at McGill was the appointment of David Landsborough Thomson to his staff in 1928. Thomson was British trained and the son of Sir Landsborough Thomson, who served under various titles as the second secretary of the British Medical Research Council from 1919 to 1957. David Thomson had studied geology and zoology at Aberdeen University. He had then been a research student at Gonville and Caius College, Cambridge, under Sir Frederick Gowland Hopkins in the Sir William Dunn Institute of Biochemistry until he received his PhD in biochemistry in 1928. During these years, he had also worked at the Marine Biological Laboratories at Millport, Plymouth, and Roscoff in Brittany, as well as at the University of Grenoble and in Zurich. He was invited to join Collip's department as lecturer in 1928 and was promoted to assistant professor the following year.

Thomson, an articulate and gifted teacher, took over all the teaching in the biochemistry department and thus freed Collip, at best a reluctant lecturer, to concentrate on the work that he most loved and was best suited for – his research. Thomson was highly literate and possessed both a photographic memory and an encyclopaedic knowledge of the scientific literature. While he was not very active in the laboratory himself, he performed the important function of keeping Collip and his staff apprised of the latest developments in other investigations. Collip called Thomson a true scholar who "commands a wider knowledge of the world literature on biological subjects than anyone else that I know."[15]

During Collip's last years at the University of Alberta, he had continued to write and conduct research on the parathyroid hormone, contributing to the elucidation of its physiological function. This work continued to occupy his interest for many years, even after the move to McGill. As Collip remarked of this line of research, "I must not forget that this is my baby and I will be expected to nurse it for some time to come." In 1928 he announced the preparation of a substance that produced a rise in blood pressure for an unusually long duration. He was able to extract this substance from a variety of tissues – including muscle, liver, ovary, and testis – using heat to pull out the principle as he had with the parathyroid hormone. He was unable to obtain the substance in a crystalline state and could not conclude whether it truly existed or whether it was an artefact of his extraction procedure. This line of work proved unfruitful and he published nothing further on it.[16]

THE HORMONES OF THE PLACENTA

In 1930 Collip's "luck" hit again, this time in the hormones of the placenta. His placental extracts brought attention to himself and to

McGill, and with it, controversy. This development had several dimensions. First, Collip was engaged in a theoretical debate about the nature and function of the active principles that he extracted from the placenta. This debate illustrates the theoretical and methodological issues that engaged sex hormone researchers of this period. Second, Collip once again found himself in the midst of an ethical debate concerning the commercial use of the results of medical science. Third, Collip was engaged in a struggle to fund his expanding research enterprise. The need for private gifts forced him and McGill officials into the troublesome business of dealing with wealthy benefactors and their potentially difficult personalities. As in the parathyroid episode, the question of priority in discovery was hotly debated, but this time in relation not only to the prestige of the investigators themselves, but also to that of their patrons and institutions. Collip used the knowledge produced in the laboratory as leverage in his negotiations with his institution and financial backers to preserve and expand his domain. To the academic institutions and private patrons, medical research became an investment opportunity, capable of transforming money into public recognition and praise.

In September 1929 Bertold P. Wiesner of the University of Edinburgh visited Collip at his laboratory and told him about his ongoing research. Wiesner, a lecturer in animal genetics, was performing a long series of experiments to examine the physiological factors relating to maternal behaviour in the rat. In this work, he had prepared extracts of the placenta with sulphosalicylic acid. He had come to believe that the placenta had two hormones. The first, which he called "Rho 1," had the effect of causing estrus and bringing immature female rats to premature puberty. The second, "Rho 11," caused luteinization and pseudo-pregnancy. Wiesner had demonstrated in what Collip called a "single but convincing experiment" that the sulphosalicylic acid extract of fresh human placenta was effective in producing premature maturity in the young rat. According to Collip, it was at Wiesner's "very urgent request" that he took up the problem of concentrating and purifying the first of these two extracts (Rho 1) and made it a subject of special study in his laboratory. Later, Collip took up work on Rho 11 as well.[17]

The two placental hormones that Collip was to isolate would bring him very different types of recognition. The hormone that caused estrus – that is, the one that had an estrogenic function – was found to have great clinical value and was developed into a commercially important therapeutic substance. The hormone that stimulated the ovary to form corpora lutea – that is, the one that had a gonadotrophic effect – had theoretical importance. Collip identified it as distinct from the biologically similar substance discovered in the anterior pituitary.[18]

The sex hormones had become the focus of intense study during the 1920s. It was known that in the female reproductive cycle, an egg is nurtured in a follicle in the ovary. The follicle then matures and releases the egg in ovulation. Then the remaining follicle tissue is transformed into the corpus luteum, which has an endocrine function of supporting pregnancy. Edgar Allen and Edward Doisy at St Louis University identified the ovarian hormone, estrin, in 1923–24. The hormone was isolated in the maturing follicles and found to have the effect of causing estrus in the female animal. The onset of estrus could be identified by a number of physical changes: the opening of the vagina; the enlargement of the uterus; and changes in the shape of the cells lining the vagina, from a columnar type to a scale-like type – a process known as cornification. Over the next ten years, many investigators isolated various forms of the estrus-causing substances; these researchers included Adolf Butenandt of Göttingen in 1929, Ernst Laqueur of Amsterdam in 1930, and Guy Marrian of the University College, London, in 1930. The substances were known by a variety of names: estrin, folliculin, oestrone, theelin, menformon, thelykinin, and pregynon.[19]

Studies of the anterior pituitary (a tiny gland located at the base of the brain) indicated that this gland served as the "conductor" of the endocrine orchestra. It regulated the action of many other endocrine glands, including the thyroid, the adrenal cortex, and the gonads. The anterior pituitary acted on the ovaries and testes by secreting gonad-stimulating, or gonadotrophic, hormones. In 1926 Bernhard Zondek of the University of Berlin and Selmar Aschheim of the Municipal Hospital of Berlin-Spandau showed that an extract of the anterior pituitary could stimulate the ovaries of immature mice to take on the appearance of puberty; that is, follicles in the ovary ripened, ovulation occurred, corpora lutea formed, and the hormone estrin was secreted from the ovary. They and other investigators discovered that this, or perhaps these, gonadotrophic principles were also present in other tissues and fluids, such as the decidua, placenta, and the blood and urine of humans and other animals in the early stages of pregnancy. This finding allowed Aschheim and Zondek to develop a test for pregnancy in 1928. One could test for the presence of gonadotrophic factors in the urine – which indicates pregnancy – by injecting a urine sample into immature mice and looking for signs of early maturity in them.

In order to succeed in this new field of research, Collip and his associates had to broaden their approach to endocrinology. In studying the hormone of the parathyroid gland and some of the other substances he had examined, Collip was able (as with insulin) to ascertain the efficacy of his extracts by observing standard physiological and biochemical responses. In his principal projects, he had been able to perform assays by using chemical tests of bodily fluids. In the case of insulin, the effect of the hormone could be determined by measuring the drop in blood glucose level, while in the case of the parathyroid hormone, its effect could be determined by measuring the rise in blood calcium. The hormones relating to growth and reproduction were more difficult to detect. Their effects were only observed in the slow changes in the shape and size of tissues and cells. As historian Merriley Borell argues, "the real pioneers of reproductive physiology were ... not the physiologists or the chemists, but the histologists who painstakingly determined the gradual changes associated with both sexual differentiation and the estrus cycle."[20]

The best test for the onset of estrus required that the experimental animal be killed and the ovaries, uterus, and vagina be sectioned and examined under the microscope for changes in shape and size of cells and tissues and for the presence of follicles and corpora lutea in the ovaries. Another test, the vaginal smear, could give a good indication of the onset of estrus without the sacrifice of the test animal. In this test, a probe was inserted into the vagina to scrape the epithelial cells lining the walls. The onset of estrus could be determined by examining the cells under the microscope and observing whether they had taken on the characteristic cornified shape.

Collip began his studies by using Wiesner's extraction method, treating fresh human placentas with sulphosalicylic acid. He found that it was difficult to remove the residual sulphosalicylic acid and to purify the extract further. Wiesner had told Collip that he had had no success in making extracts with alcohol or acetone, but Collip attempted preliminary trials with these solvents. He discovered that extracts made with either acetone or faintly acidulated alcohol were invariably potent. Because of this, he decided to abandon Wiesner's method and instead develop an extract based on the use of acetone or alcohol. The yield he obtained was very small, in the range of one milligram of extract per kilogram of original placenta.[21]

An important breakthrough in the work came about through serendipity. Control immature animals were placed in the same cages as the test immature animals injected with extract. Collip noted that certain of the control animals were inexplicably undergoing estrus along with the test animals. Since some fluid almost always leaked from the site of the injection and since the rats were given to licking each other's coats, he speculated that the hormone could perhaps be administered by mouth. He mixed the extract with lean ground meat and fed it to the rats. Indeed, the rats came into estrus prematurely. This chance observation and quick thinking pointed the way to an important characteristic of this new principle – that it was orally active, a property that was highly desirable in something that would be used for medical therapy. This discovery was particularly gratifying to Collip because of his many failed attempts to use insulin and parathyroid hormone orally.[22]

By February 1930, Collip felt sufficient confidence in his results that he published a series of preliminary papers in the *Canadian Medical Association Journal* and placed a short note in *Nature*. He announced that he had found that extracts of the placenta caused immature rats and mice to mature early and that the extracts were orally active. He also reported on the clinical trials he had conducted in collaboration with A.D. Campbell at the Royal Victoria and Montreal General hospitals. Campbell was in the Department of Gynaecology and Obstetrics at McGill. Collip and Campbell tested the preparation on patients with delayed puberty, dysmenorrhea, amenorrhea, *Metropathia hemorrhagica*, menopause, toxemia of pregnancy, certain neurological and psychiatric cases, and thyroid dysfunction. They reported definite and encouraging results.[23]

To supply this research program, placentas were collected from maternity wards at the Sisters of the Misericordia Hospital and the Royal Victoria Maternity Hospital. In 1926 the Royal Victoria Hospital had amalgamated with the Montreal Maternity Hospital, creating a splendid new women's hospital with 213 beds, 100 cribs, and state-of-the-art facilities.[24] Collip's associate in this work, Walter W. Chipman, in 1929 was just retiring as professor of obstetrics and gynaecology at McGill and as director of the Women's Pavilion at the Royal Vic. In his retirement, Chipman continued to serve on the boards of the university and the hospital and for many years visited the hospital almost daily. Collip relied on colleagues in gynaecology such as Chipman. In addition to being his collaborators on clinical trials, they supplied him with the raw materials for research. Research in the sex hormones required steady and abundant supplies of such things as human placentas, pregnancy urine, and other materials associated with human reproduction. Gynaecological clinics were a rich source. Nelly Oudshoorn argues that since laboratory researchers had to depend on gynaecologists to gain access to these supplies, the research questions they chose reflected the practical interests of their clinician partners. This created a strong orientation towards problems of human female reproductive disorders. Collip's interest in the clinical use of the hormone in these sorts of ailments reflects the clinicians' considerations outlined by Oudshoorn as well as his own long-standing interest in finding practical therapeutic applications for his extracts.[25]

The discovery had consequences beyond the laboratory. For the McGill administrators, Collip's achievement was a testimony to their efforts at rebuilding the good name of McGill's medical school. Martin and Currie were actively involved in presenting the extract to the public and in negotiating its development with commercial firms. In addition to the prestige such a product could bring to the university, it also held out the promise of financial rewards, both from the royalties generated by the sales of the product and from benefactors who might be inspired by the success of the work to contribute to McGill. Because McGill was privately funded and because the Depression was beginning to have an affect on the finances of the university, the matter of promoting the extract was pressing. To the warrior, Currie, scientific discovery was analogous to a contest in which many could play but only one could win. To the scientific men, Martin and Collip, discovery was only the small final step in a larger enterprise to which many workers had freely made contributions over many years. This notion of scientific work was to come into conflict with the goal of developing a product for commercial manufacture.

The university issued a press release on 12 February announcing that "a remarkable discovery" had been made. "Everyone at McGill University rejoices exceedingly that complete success has rewarded the long and patient efforts of Professor Collip and his capable assistants in the Bio-Chemistry Laboratories of our Medical School." The substance was characterized as "a remedial agent for certain feminine disorders." While the investigators were reticent about pronouncing on the full value of the new product, they reported that the few clinical tests done so far had shown remarkable results and posited that "the field of usefulness for this drug can hardly be over estimated." Perhaps because Collip was particularly wary after his experience with Hanson, the press release noted that the discovery had been based upon Wiesner's work. Martin wrote, "It seems to be a genuinely good thing and while we are a little bit reserved as to the ultimate benefits it certainly looks as though it was a great opportunity for further investigation in Therapeutics."[26]

Others in the field took notice. Fuller Albright, the Harvard endocrinologist, wrote to congratulate Collip on his discovery. Albright had become interested in the problem the previous summer when he had spent a few days with Zondek and Aschheim in Berlin, and with Wiesner during an Atlantic crossing. Albright offered either to send an associate or to come himself to Montreal to spend some time learning about Collip's method. Members of the public responded as well. Patients wrote to McGill asking for the new medicine, only to be told that it was not yet ready for distribution.[27]

During the winter and spring of 1930, Collip continued with his attempts to isolate and identify his preparation. In his initial publications, he argued that his extract was distinct from the previously identified hormone estrin that was known to be found in the placenta. Estrin was characterized by its ability to produce estrus in a castrated female rat. It was known to occur in the ovary, placenta, amniotic fluid, and the urine of pregnancy. Since one of the properties of estrin was that it was soluble in ether, Collip subjected his fraction to several washes with ether to remove all the estrin.

At first Collip toyed with the hypothesis that his product was the same as the ovary-stimulating principle that other investigators had isolated from the anterior pituitary, but he increasingly became convinced otherwise. One of the key characteristics distinguishing estrin from the anterior pituitary principle was estrin's effectiveness in both normal and castrated animals. In contrast, the anterior pituitary hormone was only effective in animals with ovaries; that is, the anterior pituitary hormone caused the phenomena of estrus through stimulating the action of the ovaries, causing them to grow in size and release estrin. Collip's extract was like the anterior pituitary hormone in that it was ineffective in the castrated animal, but Collip suspected a difference between them in that, unlike the pituitary hormone, his was orally active and could survive treatment with the digestive enzymes. Working on the assumption that the placental and pituitary fractions were not the same, he tried to develop a technique to assay the presence of one or the other principles in the blood as a means of determining its properties. As was typical, Collip used immense quantities of raw material to create his extracts. In March Collip reported to Henry Dale that he had made all the extract up to that point by himself and had used "something like a ton and a half of human material."[28]

By April, Collip's clinical work was proceeding well but he was concerned that he had been giving too much attention to it at the expense of his work on the chemistry of the extract. In a paper submitted to the *Canadian Medical Association Journal*, he provided the first detailed description of his method of preparing the extract. In the same paper, he also proposed the name "Emmenin" for the product, a name suggested by A.B. Macallum in reference to its property of promoting menstruation, that is, acting as an emmenogogue. Collip reported that he had encountered some difficulties with his biological assay. He complained to Martin that "the rat test has pretty well blown up due to some seasonal or other factor." Rats as young as four weeks began to show spontaneous estrus, and Collip found that he had to use much younger ones for testing. In the meantime, he decided to appraise the strength of the extracts for clinical use by measuring the grams of original placenta per cubic centimetre of extract, since he trusted the reliability of his methods of processing over the more variable rat test.[29]

PREGNANT WITH TROUBLE:
SCIENCE, COMMERCE, AND PHILANTHROPY

By early February, Collip and the McGill administrators began confer-
ring with a number of pharmaceutical companies to arrange for the
manufacture of the placental hormone. The first they contacted was,
not surprisingly, Eli Lilly & Company. Lilly's president indicated that
he considered this discovery very promising and was interested in cooperating with McGill in its development. An agreement was made
with Lilly for the exclusive rights to manufacture and distribute the
product on the American market. The head of a leading Montreal firm,
Charles E. Frosst & Company, also called upon McGill's principal,
hoping to persuade him to allow his company to manufacture the preparation. The McGill group negotiated with Burroughs Wellcome about
the manufacture of the product in Britain. The pharmaceutical company that contributed most to the development of Collip's extract,
however, was the small Montreal firm Ayerst, McKenna & Harrison.
Ayerst was eventually the only firm to invest heavily in the development of the product and to manufacture it successfully. A preliminary
application was made for a Canadian patent, with the plan that the
rights would be turned over to McGill, just as had been the case with
insulin at Toronto. The McGill group authorized Ayerst to manufacture the extract in Canada for distribution throughout the British Empire, exclusive of Great Britain and Ireland. Later, the agreement with
Lilly and the negotiations with Burroughs Wellcome failed because, according to McGill officials, the firms were unable, or perhaps unwilling, to put the product on the market at a reasonable price. When this
happened, Ayerst picked up the rights to distribute in the United States
and Britain.[30]

Ayerst, McKenna & Harrison was a young firm. Incorporated in
1924, it had commenced business early in 1925. The company's
founders, W.A.S. Ayerst, W.J. McKenna, William Harrison, and Hugh
McPherson, had gained years of experience in the pharmaceutical manufacturing field working at Charles Frosst. The new company distinguished itself by its strong commitment to research. One of its earliest
undertakings was to set up the first commercial biological laboratory in
Canada, and the first work of this laboratory was to test and standardize cod liver oil. Four years later, Ayerst produced the first concentrated
cod liver oil as a result of its research work. A portion of the initial
profits from this product was set aside for research and development.[31]

Ayerst invested heavily in the development of Emmenin. The firm expanded its laboratory work, its staff, and its animal colony, and also
added a control laboratory for the new chemical assays on estrogens.

As J.C. Simpson, Martin's successor as dean, said later, the firm did the "spade work" to develop Emmenin and establish a market for it. The extent to which the company was involved in the research and development of the product is indicated in the memoirs of Magnus Pyke, the chemist perhaps best known as a television personality later in life. Pyke, then a student at McGill's Macdonald College, worked in the small research laboratory at Ayerst, McKenna & Harrison during the summer of 1932, working closely with Collip on several aspects of the development of Emmenin. Most memorable to Pyke was his work in determining the biological activity of samples of Emmenin. This required that he inject the extract into immature female mice and perform vaginal smears on them, rubbing cells off their vaginas with the tip of a probe every day and examining the cells under a microscope. He recalled, "My duties were bizarre to say the least ... I must have taken smears from thousands of mice during the course of that summer and brought hundreds to a state of precocious sexual maturity." He remembered assisting in the preparation of the extract "made in various ways thought up by Professor Collip, and purified by more and more elaborate procedures." Also strongly impressed in his memory was the image of the "gruesome specimens" of placentas arriving from the maternity hospital in milk churns.[32]

In the midst of these developments, Collip came up against private philanthropist Thomas Bassett Macaulay, a prominent member of the Montreal business community. Robertson Macaulay and his son, Thomas Bassett, were the enterprising father and son duo who managed the Sun Life Assurance Company of Montreal for sixty years. The father, Robertson, was described as "a true Highland Scot in temperament ... a balanced mixture of the practical and the visionary." He had been born in Aberdeenshire and had come to Canada to seek his fortune at the age of twenty-one.[33] The Macaulays, known for their aggressive risk-taking style of business, helped to make Sun Life the largest life insurance company in Canada, with markets in many parts of the world. During the period after the First World War, Sun Life, like other life insurance companies, began to view an improvement of public health as being in the interests of both the insurer and the insured. The firm thus began to make contributions to medical care and research. During the 1927 typhoid epidemic in Montreal, Sun Life set up free clinics that allowed some fifty thousand people to receive inoculations.[34]

T.B. Macaulay took over the management of the firm from his father in 1906 and led it to even greater success. While he had been born and raised in Canada, the younger Macaulay had apparently maintained an interest in the welfare of Scotland. On his model experimental farm in Hudson Heights, Quebec, he worked on projects to improve wastelands of the Scottish islands and highlands. After the stock market crash in 1929, however, Macaulay and Sun Life faced the financial repercussions of Macaulay's daring investment practices. During this troubled time, Collip and the McGill group came up against this "finance czar." Macaulay had generously endowed the Animal Breeding Research Department of the University of Edinburgh, supporting the work of Wiesner and his associate, F.A.E. Crew. Macaulay himself had been responsible for introducing Wiesner to Collip when Wiesner had visited Montreal. Subsequently, Macaulay was appalled when it began to look as though the McGill scientists were about to gain all the glory for the work initiated by Wiesner and Crew.[35]

President Currie wrote to C.F. Martin, concerned that Macaulay's attitude to Collip's success was "rather pregnant with trouble." In Currie's opinion, Macaulay simply did not understand, or perhaps was unwilling to accept, how credit was accorded in the scientific world:

There is no doubt that Collip, and Collip alone, cut the Gordian knot. In most of these scientific successes there is one man who finds the last difficult solution. There are many who make contributions but it usually remains for one to make the startling discovery. In this field in which Collip has been successful the same story prevails. Japanese and French and Germans and others have worked on the problem. No doubt the Edinburgh authorities carried it on, but it was Collip who brought it to its final, startling, successful end.[36]

Even Macaulay's private physician was enlisted to visit Collip and tell him that there was some indication that the Edinburgh group had taken a "critical and threatening" attitude to the developments at McGill. He also told Collip that Macaulay was of the opinion that McGill should share its profits with Edinburgh. When Currie heard of this, he brusquely told Collip that he was "to do nothing of the sort." Macaulay then approached Currie himself and voiced his objections to the profits he thought McGill was now set to make. He even intimated that perhaps the university's fund-raising campaign was unnecessary, now that it could use Emmenin profits to build its gymnasiums and student residences.[37]

Currie dismissed these protests. Satisfied that Collip had given Wiesner and Crew every possible credit, he speculated that all this trouble had arisen because the Edinburgh scientists had tried to flatter their benefactor. He had heard that Crew had written to Macaulay telling him that Collip's success was the first tangible result of Macaulay's endowment to Edinburgh. Macaulay had admitted to Currie that he had been much criticized for making his gift to Edinburgh rather than McGill, and Currie charged, "His vanity has been wounded because he put his money on the wrong horse when he backed Edinburgh; although he backed a good horse." Currie even reported that Macaulay had told him that he felt he had more to do with Emmenin than Collip did, since his money had made Wiesner's work possible in the first place and it had been he who had then introduced Wiesner to Collip. Currie complained to Martin:

I don't know what is the matter with Mr. Macaulay – and yet I do, though. Perhaps you attended the Sun Life banquet which marked his fifty years' association with the Company. Only yesterday Jack Cook mentioned it when we were chatting and said he was never more disgusted than he was with the way the old man lapped up the flattery that was heaped upon him that night. Edinburgh (and all credit to them) have made him feel that he is one of the world's great inspirations to scientific work, and he is willing to pay for it. I know he is going to be pounced upon by the other governors of the University and made to give quite as much.[38]

As a way of placating Macaulay, Currie made him a governor of McGill and gave him an honorary LLD in 1930. That same year he was also conferred an honorary doctorate at Edinburgh University and Aberdeen University. Currie wrote, "Edinburgh has tickled his vanity to such an extent that I believe he is raising his grant of $125,000 to $4,000,000 to found there the Macaulay Institute." As it turned out, that year Macaulay indeed donated a further £3,000 to Edinburgh for research in sex physiology and £1,500 for a rat house; he also created the Macaulay Laboratory in the Institute of Animal Genetics, the Macaulay Research Fellowship, and even the Macaulay Lectureship in Animal Genetics, of which Wiesner was the first holder.[39]

Collip in the meantime had been forging ahead with his scientific work, but he could not help but be very disturbed by this situation. He reported to Martin that he had been "plugging along at full speed without a break and [was] ... just about ready for a holiday and change." As for the issue of giving credit, he declared, "Personally I have a clear conscience as far as doing justice to Wiesner is concerned." After his experience with Hanson in the parathyroid hormone episode, Collip took great care to credit his predecessors in this work, particularly Wiesner. In several of his publications, he made prominent mention of Wiesner's visit to his laboratory and of Wiesner's "urgent request" that Collip try his hand at the isolation of the placental factors. In a paper submitted in April 1930, Collip stated explicitly that his work "may be said to be built upon and to be [the] outcome of the earlier work of Wiesner and his collaborators." Collip admitted to Martin that he was aware that the Edinburgh investigators might have been hurt that he had withheld his method of extraction from them until April, but he assured him that he was intending to send them a copy of his second paper, which contained a detailed description of the method. He was anxious that he not be "in any way to be the means of possible discord" between the two universities. For this reason, he asked Martin to visit the group in Edinburgh to determine what their feelings were in the matter.[40]

A SECOND PRINCIPLE

In the laboratory, it became apparent to Collip that some other principle was present in the placenta that had yet to be accounted for. He observed that when a crude version of the extract was administered by injection rather than orally, it caused both the formation of corpora lutea and the phenomena of estrus. However, when a purified preparation of Emmenin was given orally, no corpora lutea appeared. His observation fit in with the theories recently proposed by Wiesner and also by Aschheim and Zondek: that two different principles acted on the ovary, one that stimulated the formation of follicles and caused estrus, and another that caused the formation of corpora lutea. Other investigators argued that the two functions were caused by one hormone and that the response of the ovary depended on how high the dosage was.

To prepare Emmenin, Collip first treated the pulped placental tissue with acetone or alcohol to begin extracting the active principle. Next, the solution was filtered and concentrated. Then, it was treated with 85 percent alcohol. Emmenin remained dissolved in the alcohol while other materials were precipitated out. When Collip worked up the residue from this precipitation, he discovered that it contained a second principle. He termed this second principle the "anterior-pituitary-like substance" because it produced corpora lutea in the immature female rat and caused an increased rate of growth in the seminal vesicle and prostate gland of immature male rats. This substance also differed from Emmenin in that it was not effective through oral administration.

The secretary of the Faculty of Medicine, J.C. Simpson, cabled Martin in England on May 20: "Confidential. Collip working with residue from Emmenin finds second hormone which may be identical Asheim Zondeck [sic] principle in Europe. Causes luteinization and hypertrophy of ovaries and hypertrophy and stimulation of seminal vesicles and prostate looks like a clean up."[41]

Thus, it appeared that there were three hormones in the placenta. The first, estrin, caused the phenomena of estrus in both normal and castrated female rats and had a slight activity when administered orally. The second, the fraction that Collip called Emmenin, was soluble in 85 percent alcohol and had similar effects to estrin except that it was not effective in castrated animals and was orally active. The third, the anterior-pituitary-like substance (APL), was insoluble in 85 percent alcohol and, while also estrogenic, had the added effect of causing luteinization. Collip hypothesized that Emmenin and APL corresponded to the two ovary-stimulating hormones described by Wiesner and by Zondek and Aschheim in pregnancy urine and the anterior pituitary.

STANDING ON A HIGHER PLANE: THE QUESTION OF PATENTS

The question of whether or not to patent medical products was hotly debated during this period. Although the American medical community was more open to the idea of medical patents than the British, even many prominent American researchers questioned its appropriateness. Critics were particularly concerned that patents would be used to block research in certain areas. They also argued that taking out patents was inconsistent with the ideals of science, which stipulated that knowledge was to be freely contributed to a common pool. Harvard physiologist W.B. Cannon stated in 1935:

The evils of patenting substances which may be essential for further advance in biology or which may be of therapeutic value and therefore not to be exploited for the benefit of manufacturers are clear enough. It seems to me utterly wrong also that someone who comes along and who does a final job, or even fails to contribute at all to the progress of research, can take out a patent on the product of many investigators and put himself into a position to make trouble for others who want to work in the field.[42]

The British government had held a particularly ambivalent attitude towards regulating therapeutic products, especially in comparison with the German and American governments. Unlike Germany and the United States, where governmental testing was provided as early as the late nineteenth century with the development of the diphtheria antitoxin, it was not until after the First World War that the British government started to regulate the production of Salvarsan for the treatment of syphilis, and only in 1925 that the Therapeutic Substances Act was passed, providing the government with standards and enforcement guidelines for the testing of chemical and biological products. Jonathan Liebenau argues that the activities of the British Medical Research Council (MRC) on insulin served as a model for later relations between the MRC and the pharmaceutical industry. The MRC officials were intensely interested in insulin in 1922 because they wanted to bring the important product to Britain, control its production, and prevent improper commercial exploitation. Liebenau notes that the British MRC was reluctant to accept the offer of the insulin patent rights from the University of Toronto for two reasons: first, they feared that the patents would be so inadequate that there would be grave difficulties in supervising and controlling manufacture; and second, the council was hesitant to accept foreign standards. Sir Walter Fletcher, secretary of the MRC, expressed serious doubts about the appropriateness of the MRC being involved in patenting, but agreed that the MRC's laboratories should conduct the research into standardizing the preparation. H.W. Dudley and H.H. Dale, biochemists and members of the senior staff, more pragmatically saw the need for the MRC to serve as a facilitator of commercial production. The MRC accepted the offer of the insulin patent but with the provision that the council not be obligated to defend the patent. The council licensed manufacturers, tested batches, coordinated clinical trials, and conducted research into methods of lowering costs of production and standardization. It also helped to protect the British industry from imported insulin. In doing this work, the MRC faced fierce criticism. Its regulation of research was called an unwarranted interference in the progress of science, and its involvement in patenting was challenged as leading to the commercialization of science. Liebenau argues that the MRC's work in later years was influenced by the difficulties it had experienced with insulin production and by the fact that, after 1925, it no longer had the incentive of fighting for the passage of the Therapeutic Substances Act. The effect was that the MRC kept a greater distance from manufacturers, as would be the case when penicillin was produced during the Second World War.[43]

By 1930, when the question of Emmenin arose, the British MRC had taken a stronger position against medical patents. Since the discovery of insulin, one of the major developments in therapeutics had been the production of vitamin D by ultraviolet irradiation, a method devised by Henry Steenbock at the University of Wisconsin in 1924. Steenbock's university had set up the Wisconsin Alumni Research Foundation (WARF) in 1925 to hold and manage the Steenbock patents and later other patents taken out by Wisconsin faculty members. Over the succeeding decades, WARF was criticized by other researchers for its aggressive style of patent management, which had as its primary goal the creation of a large endowment for research. Through the 1930s and 1940s, the foundation was widely condemned for misusing its patent ownership to set up monopolies to protect the state's dairy industry. The MRC was particularly anxious about this development because the production of vitamin D by irradiation had also been developed in its own laboratories, supported by public monies and freely published. There was considerable doubt about the validity of the American patent: first, because it was drawn in such wide terms that it covered many subsequent valuable applications; and second, because it was claiming the rights to a natural process, that is, the action of the ultra-violet light of the sun. Nevertheless, British manufacturers preferred to pay royalties to the American foundation rather than risk litigation. Furthermore, British researchers felt forestalled in conducting research in the area. The fallout from WARF's management of the vitamin D patent was to become important in the MRC's response to Emmenin.[44]

For Walter Fletcher, the MRC's most pressing concern was to ensure that patents would not become an obstacle to further research by other scientists. The council policy, stated first in 1928 and reaffirmed in 1931, was that it would accept patent rights where it was deemed in the public interest, whether to allow for the development of a discovery or to prevent exploitation. It would, however, "not countenance patenting in any case where, by reason of an attempt to cover unexplored ground or otherwise, this step seems likely to hamper the freedom of research or to discourage further investigation." The council recommended that patents on medical products be abolished or at least be dedicated to a public body on a compulsory basis. Fletcher told Collip that the MRC had been funding Wiesner's research for some time and that in recent months Wiesner had reported that he would soon be able to supply two of the placental substances for extensive clinical trials. There was no proposal to take out patents on those preparations, but Fletcher had some concern that Wiesner's trials and use of the product might be hampered by the commercial considerations of others: "I have quite frankly mentioned the possibilities of difficulty for us which the situation seems to include, because I believe that you will sympathize with [our] point of view. I would at the same time assure you that we are no less anxious that the results of your own work should be brought, by whatever means may seem best, to practical application in this country and elsewhere."[45]

Henry Dale added, "With whatever firm, or firms, in this country you make an arrangement, I hope that any licence will include a clause making it clear that they have no right to interfere with the production of your product for purposes of investigation."[46]

Charles Martin travelled to Britain in May, accompanied by Walter Chipman. Their first stop was in Edinburgh to meet with Crew and Wiesner to try to determine their position on Emmenin. Martin reported back that he liked the Edinburgh scientists and found that "there is no foundation for worry about Crew & Wiesner – they were both most cordial & frank." He added that they were having difficulties reproducing Collip's experiments, but as Martin had confidence in Collip's abilities, he thought that it must be a problem with their technique. He added reassuringly, "One thing is certain they admire [Collip], his work – his appreciation of their efforts & are only too anxious to see him get all possible benefit."[47]

Martin and Chipman then travelled to London to meet with the officials of the Medical Research Council. Currie was anxious to maintain cordial relations with the council, and Collip, too, wanted to ensure that McGill would not patent or license in Britain unless the British MRC approved. The personal connection between David Thomson, Collip's associate, and his father, Sir Landsborough Thomson, then second secretary of the MRC, must have made the importance of good relations even more clear. Simpson, secretary of the Faculty of Medicine, wired Martin in London with the suggestion that he go a reasonable way to meeting the wishes of council officials in the negotiations. Martin, who counted Walter Fletcher a personal friend, went with Chipman to meet with Fletcher and Dale in the council offices and later at Claridge's Hotel. Martin had learned in Edinburgh that there was considerable concern arising in Britain about difficulties that researchers were encountering with patents issued in North America and Germany. He wrote to Currie, "There is much feeling here on this subject owing to Steenbock of Madison having 'collared' the patent on 'all irradiated foods' – rather shocking I think & and not a credit to the University." Martin reported that both Fletcher and Dale deplored the practice of universities holding patents as "a bad principle for academic institutions, and as a very bad example for the future." Fletcher and Dale had told him that they had accepted the patent for insulin only because no law had existed in Britain that allowed them to standardize the preparation legally. Since the 1925 Therapeutic Substances Act, however, they felt it was unnecessary for a university to protect itself with patents. In fact, the council stopped paying the renewal fees on its patents for insulin after 1931, allowing them to lapse, since it deemed the patents no longer necessary for ensuring the quality of the product. Fletcher and Dale indicated that they would find it a relief if McGill would "stand on a higher plane" and agree to forego a patent. The MRC officers were amenable to McGill receiving royalties without a patent and to the idea of giving Lilly and Ayerst a period of exclusive rights to allow them a fair start in the market. They hoped, however, that at the end of the period Collip would send his formula to the MRC for safekeeping and to ensure the control of its use in research and manufacturing. Martin and Chipman agreed: "After hearing all the evidence, we doubt if it is wise for McGill to issue a patent, and we would certainly have a better academic standing among our British colleagues if we refrained." Martin added that Dale and Fletcher "spoke of Collip's personal academic attitude in the very highest terms."[48]

In the end, in deference to the wishes of the British MRC, the McGill group decided not to patent the product. Martin and Collip, as English Canadian medical scientists of this era, were anxious to adhere to the code of honour set out by the British medical and scientific community. They felt that sufficient protection could be given the pharmaceutical firms cooperating with them by simply allowing them a period of exclusive licence during which they could gain a head start on their competitors.[49] It is also true that the British stance in this matter was not simply one of principle but also included some self-interest. The MRC was actively protecting a piece of scientific work that it had invested in. This episode reflects the conflicts engendered by the growing importance of commerce to medical science. In one respect, the McGill group was anxious to exploit the commercial potential of their laboratory finding; this fit with Currie's view of scientific work as a horse race in which the whole prize goes to the winner. In another respect, Collip and Martin were aware that any accomplishment in science is founded upon the work of others; in this scheme, it was unfair to allow someone who had only completed the final link in the chain to reap all the rewards.

CONTINUING RESEARCH

By the summer, the problems in the laboratory and the troubles with Macaulay were weighing heavily on Collip and he felt ready for a holiday. He remarked to Martin that he was having so much difficulty with things going wrong and was "in such a state" that he felt he had to "clear out for a breathing space." He spent the summer in Britain with his family but made his first stop at Edinburgh. Upon landing, he immediately met with Wiesner and Crew at his hotel. Delighted to receive a warm welcome from them, he spent a further week in Edinburgh and Aberdeen before proceeding south to London, where he met with Henry Dale and Walter Fletcher.[50]

Instead of taking a holiday as planned, Collip immediately took the opportunity to start up his research at the National Institute for Medical Research (NIMR) at Hampstead, the MRC's central laboratories. By July he was able to report to Martin that he had been hard at work for a month working up over a hundred kilograms of placentas. He commented that he was getting enough biological assays finished "to cheer me up in great style." Although he was unable to prepare the highly purified product that he had also sought to make in February, he was delighted to find that his Hampstead preparation was equal to or better than any he had made before. He happily noted, "And as I have been working with a different colony of rats which have not as yet learned the bad habits of Montreal rats, I feel very gratified indeed."[51]

Collip's theory about the identity of Emmenin changed as his work progressed. Until April he had been certain that his product was one of the ovary-stimulating hormones that Wiesner had isolated. While in England, he began to suspect that Emmenin was some new hormone with characteristics somewhere between those of estrin and Wiesner's Rho I and Rho II complex. In fact, he recognized that its properties were even closer to those of estrin than to those of the ovary-stimulating principle of the anterior pituitary. He wrote to Martin: "I was a bit worried about this for a time but I cannot believe that I have been working with oestrin." He was confident that he had taken every precaution to remove estrin with washes of ether and that he had managed to exclude estrin as far as possible with known methods. He admitted that he could have presented this information more clearly in his first paper had he known the results of the more recent work but he had been anxious to publish his method in detail as early as possible so that his claims could be tested by others. Finally, he reported that he had managed to squeeze in a holiday despite himself: "In spite of all my worries I have managed to enjoy the change. Mrs. Collip and the children have had a wonderful time in London too. We have taken in nearly all the theatres and on the weekends we have gotten out to the sea or country."[52]

At the end of August, Collip and his family finished their British stay and set sail for Montreal. He left his precious placental extracts behind, entrusted to the care of Henry Dale, whom he asked to arrange for a clinical trial. Unfortunately, others at the NIMR were not as confident of the value of these extracts as Collip was. A.S. Parke, another endocrine researcher at the institute at the time, later recalled the events he dubbed "the affair of the Collip cocktail":

The extract, which filled a row of half-gallon bottles and occupied valuable space in the Institute's small cold room, was left behind by Collip for clinical trial, the recommended dose, if I remember rightly, being 80 ml twice a day by mouth. It proved to be an embarrassing legacy. Sir Henry, then Director of the Institute, probably torn between a desire to liberate his cold room and reluctance to arrange clinical trials of such a nebulous product, passed the problem to the newly formed Sex Hormones Committee.[53]

Parkes was instructed to call an emergency meeting of the committee to determine the fate of the extract. The committee members cautiously agreed to do some laboratory tests on it and discovered that the "brew" contained about 60 per cent alcohol. "At its next meeting the Committee solemnly reported 'that no reliable clinical trials can be performed without the most thorough investigation of the effect of control preparations of alcohol.'" Parkes concluded, "So far as I know, the written record does not state what happened to the row of bottles in the cold room."[54]

By the latter part of 1930, Collip was obtaining more data linking Emmenin with estrin. Earlier, he had felt that Emmenin's ineffectiveness in castrated animals was proof that his extract was not the same as estrin. He was finding, however, that Emmenin could be made effective in adult castrated animals if taken in very large doses and in immature animals that were freshly castrated. Furthermore, studies failed to find any anatomical change in the ovaries of rats treated with Emmenin, as would be expected if it were an ovary-stimulating substance. By April 1932, Collip had concluded that Emmenin was not an ovary-stimulating substance as he had originally thought, but rather an estrogenic agent.

Collip's colleague and doctoral student J.S.L. Browne had made a parallel study. Browne had worked up the estrin in the ether washes and had prepared a crystalline compound from it. Collip and Browne determined that this substance was identical in gross chemical and physiological properties to the Emmenin fraction. They had to conclude, therefore, that Emmenin was a form of estrin and that it existed in two configurations, one that was soluble in ether and had been removed in the ether washes, and a second, the original fraction they had called Emmenin, that was not soluble in ether. The portion that was ether-insoluble could be rendered ether-soluble by hydrolysis under high pressure. Collip announced that Emmenin could also be prepared from the urine of pregnant animals. It became apparent that his product was similar to, or possibly identical with, the estrogenic substances produced by several other investigators in recent years. Among those were the theelol of Edward Doisy at St Louis, the trihydroxy oestrin isolated in 1930 by Guy Marrian at University College, London, and the similar compound prepared by Adolf Butenandt in Göttingen in 1929.[55]

Collip's study of his other fraction, the anterior-pituitary-like hormone of the placenta, proved to be fruitful. APL had many features in common with the ovary-stimulating hormones of the pituitary, but there were also important differences between them. In pursuing the questions of whether or not the placental and pituitary principles were identical and how many ovary-stimulating hormones there were, Collip was drawn into the study of the hormones of the anterior pituitary itself. This field would occupy him for the remainder of his years in the laboratory, and he would make important contributions to it. Significantly, Collip and his group were able to demonstrate that the placental APL was indeed a different principle from the pituitary substance.

In later years, Martin remarked that he was satisfied with their decisions about the commercial development of Emmenin. "Thank God we have never patented the thing, if for no other reason than that it has

pleased Fletcher and the other members of the Medical Research Council." The decision not to patent, however, led to some difficulties for
their commercial partner. The older ethical code of medical scientists
became more and more difficult to uphold in the face of science's
increasing involvement with the competitive and profit-oriented field of
drug manufacture. By 1932 the growing understanding of the chemical
composition of Emmenin made it possible for other manufacturers to
prepare the product. McGill had more than a financial stake in the success of the product; it also had an interest in ensuring that anything
sold under the name of Emmenin met Collip's standards of efficacy. A
market for the product had been created because it had been shown to
be effective in several types of menstrual disorder. It was popular because it could be easily and safely given by mouth. Although other
forms of estrin had some oral activity, they were generally injected
parenterally.[56]

Ayerst, McKenna & Harrison became particularly concerned about
protecting its investment. The firm had worked closely with McGill
and had initially obliged its collaborators by respecting their wish not
to patent Emmenin. Later, however, difficulties with one of their other
products persuaded the Ayerst directors that they had to take greater
measures to safeguard Emmenin. In October 1932 the Wisconsin
Alumni Research Foundation notified the firm that it was infringing on
a patent held by WARF for the use of copper and iron for the treatment
of anemia. This product had been available in Canada and the United
States since February 1930, and Ayerst had marketed it as "Cupron."
Then, in September 1932, Edwin Hart patented the product for WARF.
Ayerst's directors felt unable to contest the patent, not only because
they believed that the law was on the side of the foundation, but also
because Ayerst was under licence by WARF to manufacture another important product, vitamin D. McKenna explained the situation as the
directors saw it: "If this Foundation cancelled our license on vitamin
D, it would mean a severe financial loss to us, in fact, we would be
obliged to withdraw certain preparations from the market, on which
we have spent considerable money since 1923." McKenna urged Martin to allow the company to protect its investment in Emmenin, arguing
that his experience in the commercial field had taught him that unless
suitable copyrights were taken out, it was only a matter of time before
some American company would gain the exclusive rights to the product. He warned that such an occurrence would deter manufacturers
from investing time and effort in the development of a product; their
work could be so easily jeopardized by those who had put no investment of their own into a product, but simply knew how to make the
law work in their favour.[57]

Martin was sympathetic to McKenna's concerns because he recognized that the firm had invested more money than it could reasonably hope to get back for quite some time and therefore it deserved some protection. Moreover, he feared that other companies might produce Emmenin without consulting Collip and that their versions of the product might reflect badly on McGill. While no patent rights were possible, McGill agreed to give the firm the exclusive rights to the trade name Emmenin, first in Canada and the United States and later in Britain as well, with the condition that the method of manufacture be controlled by the McGill biochemistry department. This did not limit manufacture of the product to Ayerst and its British partner, Glaxo, but it gave them the advantage of reaching the market with a product with a familiar-sounding name.[58]

In December 1934 Ayerst encountered further difficulties, this time with establishing the trade name on the American market. After acquiring the rights to market Emmenin in the United States, Ayerst set up an American subsidiary and a plant at Rouses Point in New York. In preparation for distributing Emmenin on the American market, Ayerst submitted an application to the American Medical Association (AMA) Council on Pharmacy and Chemistry for acceptance of the trade name. Approval by the council was virtually essential if a firm hoped to be successful in presenting a product to American physicians. The council, however, determined that the name Emmenin was inappropriate. According to McKenna and Harrison, the AMA representatives were opposed to the name because the council's rules stipulated that names should not be therapeutically suggestive. Instead, they suggested some name that indicated the origin of the substance, such as "placentamine." While the council representatives did not like the name Emmenin, they were willing to accept Collip's designation, since he was the discoverer, but only as the non-proprietary name. Ayerst was faced with the prospect of either having to share the name that the firm had spent four years developing a market for, or selecting a new name and starting again. McKenna pleaded to Martin that "it seems to us this course is rather drastic and, indeed, unfair." Alternately, if the council agreed to allow Ayerst to use Emmenin as its trade name, it would likely adopt another name as the non-proprietary name and Collip would be faced with the probability that his discovery would be known by some other name in the American medical literature. The firm asked Martin to apply pressure on the AMA and on the Canadian Medical Association (CMA) as well. McKenna reported that although Ayerst had not yet established permanent representation on the American market, its sales during the previous month were over 40 per cent greater in the United States than in Canada, where it had been working intensively at developing the market for some time. "This indicates something of the possibilities of the American field and the importance of consistently safeguarding the University's interest in the name under which this material is to be marketed there."[59]

Martin solicited the support of the CMA, arguing that while McGill was firmly opposed to taking out any patent, it wanted to ensure the integrity of the product by placing its manufacture and distribution in the hands of a firm in which it had confidence. He explained further that the university had been very satisfied with its part in the arrangement but recognized that Ayerst had not yet profited by it because the company had to surmount great difficulties in the manufacturing process. The name Emmenin was particularly important, not only on sentimental grounds – it had been suggested by A.B. Macallum, who had since died – but because the university would have no control over the use of the name and could not ensure the integrity of the product. The CMA responded favourably by sending a letter to the AMA asking it to reconsider the Ayerst application. However, in a final decision, Morris Fishbein of the AMA replied that his council was unable to break its own rules and that Emmenin would not be considered a satisfactory designation.[60]

Throughout its dealings with Ayerst, the McGill group found the firm to have acted honourably, not only fulfilling all its promises, but going beyond their written obligations and meeting every legitimate request made of them. In return, the success of Emmenin helped establish Ayerst as an important player in the pharmaceutical market. As one of the first orally active estrogens, Emmenin brought a great deal of interest from endocrinologists and gynaecologists. The establishment of a successful American subsidiary by a Canadian pharmaceutical company was unique and only made possible by the company's collaboration with McGill on Emmenin. The factor preventing competitors from entering into the manufacture of Emmenin was the prohibitive price of the raw materials. Ayerst was able to develop a good supply of placentas in Montreal, and when it opened its Rouses Point plant, the firm managed to arrange for a special permit to export placentas from Montreal.[61]

In the 1940s the market for Emmenin was challenged by the development of a synthetic alternative, stilbestrol, particularly the compound diethylstilbestrol (DES). The synthetic estrogen was orally active, twenty times more potent than natural estrogens, and much less expensive to produce. DES became the first widely used product for estrogen replacement therapy in treating a variety of gynaecological conditions, such as vaginitis, amenorrhea, dysmenorrhea, the symptoms of menopause, the inhibition of lactation, and – with tragic results that were only discovered later – the prevention of miscarriage. At the request of Ayerst, McGill agreed to reduce the royalties it received from 5 per cent to 2 per cent so that Ayerst could market its product more cheaply in order meet the expected competition.[62]

In addition, Ayerst's research team developed a more potent, orally active form of natural estrogen, called "Premarin." This was an even more successful product than Emmenin, and it transformed Ayerst's American arm into a large, profitable operation. The company continued to maintain its ties with McGill and Collip, and advertised on its packaging that Emmenin and Premarin had been standardized in Collip's lab. In return for using the reputations of Collip and McGill, Ayerst paid royalties towards Collip's research on both Emmenin and its own product, Premarin. In 1943 the firm was acquired by American Home Products Corporation.[63] By the end of the century, Premarin would become the top-selling prescription drug in North America, making Ayerst's successor, Wyeth-Ayerst, $1.9 billion in global sales and giving it two-thirds of the market share for menopause drugs.[64]

The fact that Collip's research produced results that were both theoretically and therapeutically significant was important to the survival of his research enterprise. The royalties from Emmenin proved to be a considerable financial boon to Collip's laboratory and to McGill. The accumulated royalties amounted to $77,743 by 1940, and the income for 1939–40 alone was $21,925. In recognition of the importance of their collaboration, Ayerst directors anonymously donated a sum of $5,000 to Collip's department in 1933. In commenting on this "modest evidence of our appreciation," they wrote, "We know that our connection with McGill University, particular through the Department of Biochemistry has been the means of creating a confidence in our firm that we would not have otherwise enjoyed." Martin regarded the news of the donation as "a bright spot in the gloomy world" and noted that "apparently there were not strings to the gift, other than that it should be used in the Department of Biochemistry."[65]

That same year, Vincent Massey donated two annual grants of $5,000 from the Massey Foundation to the work of Collip's laboratory, saying, "My wife and I have been much impressed by what we have heard of the importance of the work carried on by Dr. Collip." To Currie, the foremost value of Collip's research was its contribution to therapeutics, and this value was amply borne out by public acclaim and the accompanying financial support. Currie replied to Massey: "[Collip] is that sort of investigator who has the faculty of achieving definite results. There is much scientific investigation which is abstract. Such investigation is by no means to be condemned, nor must one always look for what may be called useful results; but I confess that, to me, there is an added pleasure when the new truth discovered can be made to serve in a positive way the well-being of mankind.[66]

ACHIEVING DEFINITE RESULTS

As the chief of a laboratory, Collip was an entrepreneur of science.[67] He had to maintain a delicate balance in negotiating among the scientific, medical, academic, and commercial worlds. The results of his research had a scientific significance as a contribution to the knowledge of the hormones of the placenta and of their relation to the other hormones of reproduction. The therapeutic value of his knowledge had considerable importance in the evolving relations among the medical community, the university, and the pharmaceutical industry. In turning his laboratory findings to commercial use, he had to try to compromise between the traditional honour-bound rules of how scientific knowledge should be disseminated and the sometimes conflicting requirements of the marketplace. Although bowing to the wishes of the British Medical Research Council in its desire to respect the conventions of the scientific and medical communities, Collip and the McGill officers also had to meet the needs of their industrial partner, since effective commercial production of Emmenin was key to public recognition and the financial stability of the research operation.

Collip's research took on a more diffuse meaning in the public eye, as a symbol of humanitarianism and a contribution to pubic welfare. It was this view of the research that drew the donations from the Macaulays and the Masseys. Collip had to navigate among the several differing meanings of biomedical knowledge and the differing sets of rules in his attempts to build and maintain his research enterprise.

5

The Great Years, 1934–1941

Collip was one of the nurserymen in our forest whom we saw rushing
from tree to tree. Fresh from the insulin tree, he hastened to the
parathyroid tree, and then was off to the sex gland trees. What he learned from
one tree he applied to the next.
Fuller Albright and Read Ellsworth, Uncharted Seas[1]

... for about 10 years everything was good fun.
J.B. Collip to Herbert Evans, 15 April 1964[2]

The 1930s have been called the great years of Collip's research career.
During this decade, he and his staff produced important contributions
to the understanding of the anterior pituitary hormones. Collip was
able to make the transition from working with one or two associates to
heading up a large laboratory group, a configuration that was to
become characteristic of modern medical research. The scientific successes of this group depended on Collip's ability to create an atmosphere of cooperation and teamwork.

The biochemistry department was a hub of activity throughout this
period. The small permanent staff of five or six was supplemented by a
constantly changing group of up to a dozen post-graduate workers,
three or four graduate students from both medical and biochemical
backgrounds, and a dozen technicians, making up to twenty to thirty
people at any particular time. Those in the department remember it as
a time of tremendous excitement and enormous productivity during
which almost two hundred papers were published. David Thomson remembered that "the department was full to overflowing, and the exhilarating wine of rapid progress animated successive batches of graduate
students." He recalled enthusiastic discussions about new ideas at all
hours of the day and night, and "rushing down to the station to put a
white-hot manuscript on the New York train" so that it could be included in the next *Proceedings of the Society for Experimental Biology
and Medicine*. At the centre of all this activity was Collip himself,
called "the Chief" by his loyal co-workers. Collip's restless, driven

nature showed itself best in his endless extractions of the tissues of tens of thousands of cattle, sheep, and hogs. His associate, Robert Noble recalled:

To meet Collip in those days one was ushered by Mr. Long (having previously established one's credentials) into a room reeking of caprylic alcohol that steamed from electrically heated garbage pails containing 10-litre flasks connected to a still through a deafening high-vacuum pump. Enormous filter funnels covered the benches and were being continuously filled from two-gallon battery jars. Conversation was impossible as Collip dashed from one tank to another until he would finally step out of the room with a small flask of brown liquid representing the concentrated activity of some hundreds of pounds of starting material. This picture became a symbol of the activity and it continued well into the night. Characteristically work went on until 1 or 2 a.m. and Collip would rarely miss a night at the lab.[3]

Although some might have assumed that the tedious work of chemical extraction was more suitably carried out by a technician, it remained Collip's great joy to do this part of the work himself. David Thomson has suggested that the long silent hours at the still may have allowed Collip to develop his best ideas. As Collip darted about his stills and funnels, adjusting the pH of one extract or filtering the precipitate of another, he smoked his trademark hand-rolled oversized cigarettes, dropping ashes on his vest as he went along. Each extract seemed to contain a slight modification, the recipe for which was jotted down in his little black notebook, much to the dismay of those who might want to duplicate his results. One long-time colleague, Abe Neufeld, recalled that Dennis O'Donovan, an Irish medical student who was doing post-graduate work in the lab at the time, would say to him, annoyed, "Abe why doesn't he tell how he makes those extracts?" The extracts Collip prepared were then put in the large refrigerators for the use of the other members of the lab.[4]

The many projects of the students and associates created a whirl of activity around Collip. O'Donovan recalled that the Chief was constantly involved in his "brewing" activities, so that he had little time to communicate with the other workers. However, Collip made it clear that each member of the department was to help the others and that all problems were to belong to the group as a whole. A key means of promoting this feeling of teamwork was the tradition of taking tea at four o'clock every day. At teatime, each member of the group learned about and ardently discussed the findings of the others. Friends and associates from other departments and universities were known to drop by for these sessions. While generally shy in social situations, Collip loved being in this atmosphere of excitement and intense activity, and he became particularly animated when new ideas caught his interest. His student J.S.L. Browne recalled: "He was quick of mind and from his questions in conversation it was apparent that his mind ran ahead of the speaker, anticipating the possible implications and ramifications of every word."[5]

New students joining the department were sometimes left to their own devices, as the Chief felt confident that they would become "absorbed into the laboratory family" through interaction with other members of the group. This was the style of training that Collip had received from Macallum at Toronto two decades before. Those who were suitably prepared fared well and came to appreciate that Collip was giving them a chance to show what they were capable of. Those who were less prepared, who expected their supervisor to tell them what to do, would find themselves assigned – more often than not – to test Collip's abstracts. Abe Neufeld, a PhD student at the University of Manitoba, remembered feeling lost after arriving in Montreal to do a year of study under Collip. Once Collip had ascertained that the newcomer had lodgings and sufficient funds, he simply deposited him at the bench he was to use and departed with the comment that he would see him later. Fortunately, Neufeld was indeed soon absorbed into the family. Through his discussions with Leonard Pugsley, Neufeld learned that some monkeys were available and he soon devised the idea of using them to study experimental diabetes. Some time later, Collip came to inquire of Neufeld's progress and learned of this plan. Neufeld recalled, "Before I had gone any further I was in Dr. Collip's office and he did most of the talking and I can say only with tremendous enthusiasm. That half hour I really learned what Dr. Collip was like – an absolute fountain of ideas, and always miles ahead of you!"[6]

Collip's daughter Barbara was very close to him and spent a lot of time in the laboratory while she was growing up. Her father would take her in with him on the weekends when she was a girl. If he were called away to the telephone, she would sometimes be left watching some brew, perhaps a little eyedropper in hand and with the instruction not to let the important stuff boil over. Later, when she was studying at McGill, she went up to the lab after class every day and waited to go home with him. During the summers, she would work there, learning how to clean glassware and perform simple tests.[7]

John Browne described the laboratory organization this way: "The 'Chief' generated the ideas and set the pace; the team members carried out the work." When Collip returned from visits to other labs, he was often particularly excited, inspired by what he had learned. While his enthusiasm was infectious, his drive and impatience with slow progress

sometimes made it difficult for others to keep up with him. Neufeld recalled having to say, "But, Dr. Collip, I have only two hands and there
are only 24 hours in a day, how can you expect me to do all that you
want to have done?" Visitors to the laboratory remembered it as a hive
of activity, with eager workers at their benches until all hours of the
night and temporary members all wanting to stay on indefinitely.[8]

Collip's second in command, David Thomson, participated less and
less in the laboratory work as the years went on, but he took on the
work of much of the teaching in the department. This contribution was
significant in that it freed Collip to pursue the research work for which
he was so much better suited. Hans Selye, a skilled anatomist and histologist trained in Prague, joined the department in 1930. Selye possessed both an MD and a PhD. He had started a one-year Rockefeller
Research Fellowship at Johns Hopkins when he became homesick and
decided to go to Canada to work with Collip, hoping that Canada
would be more European in culture. He spent the second half of his
year at McGill and went back to Prague at the conclusion of his fellowship. When Collip offered him a position as lecturer in his department,
he leapt at the opportunity and returned to Montreal permanently in
1933. Evelyn Anderson, also an MD and PhD, had come from the University of California at Berkeley to work with Collip as a National Research Council fellow; she, too, stayed on after her fellowship expired.
While Collip could only offer her a small salary, he remarked to a
Rockefeller officer that she was "worth worlds more." Rounding out
this group was a constantly changing array of post-doctoral fellows, independent investigators who attached themselves to the group with no
salary, several doctoral students, and seven or eight technicians. One of
Collip's most brilliant students was J.S.L. Browne. Browne completed
his doctorate with Collip in 1932 and went on to establish an important centre of research in clinical endocrinology at McGill.[9]

Collip's restless personality showed itself in the way he directed the
work of the laboratory. His style was, as Robert Noble described, to
" 'skim the cream off a problem' and then go quickly on to the next."
Another colleague, R.J. Rossiter, remembered Collip as possessing intense feelings and strongly held views and as always quick in thought
and action. Rossiter also characterized him as an individualist who resisted regimentation. He regarded Collip as a person of great integrity
who, even though he could be greatly upset by criticism, would continue to do what he thought to be right regardless of other people's
opinions. Browne and Denstedt described him as someone who was
apt to make decisions immediately, sometimes just to get the matter off
his mind. Once, inspired by a novel observation made by his co-worker
Hugh Long, Collip cancelled a family trip to Australia at a few hours'

notice. This characteristic carried over to his love of games, especially where a gamble was involved. It displayed itself, for example, in his enthusiasm for playing the stock market. Noble described the laboratory as sometimes seeming to be overrun with stockbrokers. Collip even had an extension telephone installed near his still so that he could take quick action on the market. His decisiveness and love of risk were complemented by his ability to know "how to cut his losses" when an occasional choice failed to pan out. His restless personality was also evident in his famous exploits behind the wheel of a car. Browne and Denstedt recalled, "When not in the lab he was happiest on the highway with Mrs. Collip by his side and, in the earlier years with the three children in the back seat, going somewhere as fast as the speed limit would permit." Noble joked that Collip's driving was legendary among friends and acquaintances and was generally considered "a form of low flying." Many students were said to have found their first car trip to a conference with the Chief more memorable than the experience of presenting their first papers.[10]

Ray Collip was well known among her husband's colleagues as a lovely, warm hostess and a patient, generous wife and mother. Married to Bert, she had to be prepared for adventures at the spur of the moment. In later years, she learned to keep a suitcase packed and ready to go, just in case. Their daughter Barbara remembers that one year her father was dismayed to learn that the reservations he thought he had for his family at Wood's Hole were somehow lost. Quickly, he found out about a cruise ship with room available but that had already left Halifax. He arrived home announcing to Ray and the children, "We're leaving tomorrow for the West Indies." Their bags hastily packed, the family boarded a train the next day for Boston to catch up with the ship. Even on the cruise, Collip's mind never strayed very far from his beloved research. He convinced the captain to have a shark caught for him. The shark's pituitary was quickly removed for his research, while its teeth went to the children as souvenirs. Collip also collected a pair of monkeys, one to be used for research, the other to be a family pet.[11]

Collip's habit of dashing from one problem to the next meant that individual subjects were perhaps not investigated with the same attention they would receive in other laboratories. M.K. McPhail, a student in Collip's lab, noted that when he later went on to Hampstead in England to do post-graduate work, he had the impression that work there was done with more thoroughness than it had been at McGill. He remembered that the McGill group had used somewhat crude techniques in photography and operative procedures and had taken less care in preparing scientific data. "This," he suggested, "undoubtedly was due in part to Collip's interest in getting the important things done and not wasting time with unnecessary details." Noble suggested that because of this many other laboratories benefited indirectly, being able to develop the McGill group's observations in greater depth.

Overall, however, those in the laboratory remembered this period as a happy and exciting time. McPhail remembered one incident when he, Browne, Pugsley, and Peter Black were headed to a scientific meeting in Philadelphia that Collip was not attending. Collip asked them if they planned to take anything for "snakebite." "This was during the days of prohibition in the U.S.A. and he advised us to take our own supplies and stay clear of 'bootlegged hootch.' We followed his advice and filled a number of amber bottles with good Scotch whisky, labeling them 'emminin.'" Every New Year's Eve, the Collips would hold a big party at their home for all the members of the lab and their families. Daughter Barbara remembers these as tremendous fun, with plenty of food and games, even a mock casino. Adults and children alike could play at roulette with rolls of new pennies. McPhail recalled: "Mrs. Collip would participate in party games quietly and effectively and her husband with such boyish exuberance, that together they made the evening a joy to everyone present. At ping pong, Dr. Collip seemed to be more often than not on the floor on his hands and knees retrieving balls. At billiards, he was much the same – he would talk, smoke, brush ashes from his clothes and make shots all at a rapid pace." The group made a tradition of toasting the pituitary hormones at this party: "May they multiply." And during the great years, they usually did.[12]

Because of Charles Martin's efforts at building the medical faculty and its research capabilities, Collip had a number of interesting colleagues in the biological and medical sciences. Biochemistry was located on the third floor of the Biological Building. On the floor above was the Department of Physiology headed by Boris Babkin, a Russian refugee and a student of Pavlov. Babkin was renowned for his work in neurophysiology, especially in relation to gastrointestinal secretion and motility. His laboratory produced important work on the hormone gastrin.[13] On the floor above Physiology was the Department of Pharmacology headed by R.L. Stehle, who was well known for his work on the posterior pituitary hormones.

In his free time, Collip was able to cultivate the friendly acquaintance of other scientists at McGill. He belonged to an informal group known as the "Greenhouse Follies Club" that met in the Biological Building's greenhouse laboratory on Monday evenings for a cold supper and a congenial discussion of scientific problems. The organizer of the group, Francis Lloyd, challenged the Follies with such problems as figuring out the mechanism of the trap in the plant "euticulare" that enabled it to catch insects. The group included such members as David Thomson, David Keys of Physics (a friend of Collip's since their Trinity days), the chemist Otto Maass, Fred Johnstone, George W. Scarth, A. Norman Shaw, and later A.S. Eve, Roney D. Gibbs, J.J. O'Neil, C.P. Martin (a physical anthropologist and the chair of anatomy), T.W.N. Cameron, V.C. Wynne-Edwards, E.F. Burr, and E.G.D. Murray, the head of the Department of Bacteriology and Immunology (known as "Joburg" to his friends for his South African origins).[14]

The school's two teaching hospitals provided other research colleagues. At the Royal Victoria Hospital, just a short walk up the street from the Biological Building, was the University Medical Clinic directed by J.C. Meakins. Meakins introduced a new emphasis on original laboratory investigation, setting up an independent research unit in which the senior appointments were made to basic scientists rather than to clinicians. C.N.H. Long, a talented physiological chemist from University College, London, was interested in the chemistry of muscular function and its relation to heart disease and anaesthesia. He completed his undergraduate studies and his MD in 1928 and left Montreal in 1933. He later became the Sterling Professor of Physiology at Yale and the dean of the Faculty of Medicine. When the Neurological Institute was completed in 1934, Wilder Penfield and William Cone moved to their new quarters. The space they vacated in the hospital was then set up as a small laboratory for endocrinology research under J.S.L. Browne. Eleanor M. Venning, who received her doctorate working with Long in 1933, assisted Browne. With an ever-increasing number of investigators and using materials drawn from the maternity hospital, Browne built an important centre of clinical research in endocrinology. Venning's contribution was her ability to develop simplified assay methods that opened up the study of the metabolites of pregnancy and the hormones of the placenta and ovary. With Browne's clinical research complementing Collip's fundamental studies, McGill was an important centre for endocrine work during the 1930s.[15]

The Montreal General Hospital was located somewhat farther away from the university, on Dorchester Street. I.M. "Rab" Rabinowitch served as pathological chemist and director of the hospital's diabetic clinic, the largest in Canada during the 1930s. He was a keen researcher and as early as 1919 set up a biochemical laboratory in a corner of the clinical laboratory. Despite the doubts of the hospital department chiefs as to the value of chemical procedures to clinical practice, Rabinowitch introduced laboratory tests for blood sugar, blood urea nitrogen, and creatinine. He had to make much of his equipment for himself, improvising with olive bottles from the kitchen to substitute for Pyrex tests tubes and borrowing the analytical balance from the Department of Biochemistry for his quantitative analyses. This laboratory grew into the department of Metabolism and then, in 1947, into the Institute for Special Research and Cell Metabolism. Rabinowitch held an appointment at McGill and lectured on pathological chemistry in Collip's department.[16]

THE ENDOCRINE GOLD RUSH: COMPETITION IN PITUITARY HORMONE RESEARCH

Hormone research was the focus of intense interest and competition among investigators during the 1930s, and this period could truly be described as an "endocrine gold rush." The hormones of the anterior pituitary were particularly interesting because the pituitary was increasingly regarded as a "master gland," responsible for regulating a vast range of bodily functions, including the control of growth and reproduction. Research centred on the problems of isolating, identifying, and determining the physiological function of the several pituitary hormones.

Collip's interest in the anterior pituitary hormones emerged from his work on the anterior-pituitary-like hormone of the placenta (APL). Considerable controversy surrounded the number and actions of the various hormones of the pituitary, and Collip was drawn into the field because he wanted to determine whether or not APL was the same as the pituitary gonadotrophins, the hormones that acted upon the gonads.[17]

An important characteristic of endocrine research was that it was carried out by investigators from many different disciplines. Historians Diana Long and Thomas Glick argue that the field of endocrinology was united by its subject matter – the secretions of the endocrine glands – rather than by its methods. Over the course of its development, the field was dominated by different disciplinary approaches in turn: first by morphology – that is, anatomy and histology – then physiology, then biochemistry, and finally molecular biology. Leading endocrine researchers of the 1920s and 1930s identified themselves variously as physiologists, anatomists, zoologists, and biochemists. When endocrine research turned to the hormones involved in growth and reproduction, it became increasingly characterized by interdisciplinary collaboration. This feature of hormone studies can be seen in the composition of the research group at Collip's laboratory as well as that of many of the other leading groups. Success required the work of a team of investigators who each brought special skills from a variety of disciplinary backgrounds.[18]

A number of laboratories around the world were engaged in research on the anterior pituitary. They produced findings rapidly, so that determining priority was sometimes difficult. Scientists from different disciplines contributed important parts of the work. The biochemist could extract and chemically characterize the active principles. The physiologist and the histologist could demonstrate the biological activity of the extract. The laboratory groups that combined the skills of the biochemist and the anatomist were particularly successful. These labs contributed key pieces of information on the hormones of the anterior pituitary, but there remained considerable controversy over the precise number and function of these hormones. While collaboration was essential to the success of these enterprises, disciplinary biases were reflected in the manner the very complex experimental results were interpreted.

The interactions of Collip's group with that of Herbert McLean Evans of the University of California, Berkeley, illustrates these tensions. These two groups achieved notable successes by mastering a new experimental system that used a hypophysectomized rat – that is, a rat from which the pituitary (also known as the hypophysis) had been surgically removed. The hypophysectomized rat could then serve almost as a *tabula rasa* in pituitary replacement therapy, the classic method of endocrine research. When the pituitary is surgically removed, growth stops and the reproductive organs, the thyroid gland, and the adrenal cortex begin to atrophy. The researcher could test the biological activity of various extracts by injecting them into this animal and determining whether they replaced any of the functions of the anterior pituitary.

The development of the technique of hypophysectomy in the rat might be said to have transformed endocrinology. Prior to the early 1920s, those who studied the function of the pituitary removed the gland from the experimental animal in a manner that produced ambiguous results. The pituitary is located at the base of the brain. To get to it, investigators entered through the cranium and lifted the brain. The problem with this method was that severe brain damage could result, leading to bleeding and death. Furthermore, it was difficult to ascertain whether the entire pituitary had been removed. Investigators therefore had difficulty determining whether or not the effects they observed were truly due to the absence of the pituitary. In 1925 Philip Smith, an anatomist and colleague of Herbert Evans, developed an alternative method of hypophysectomy in which he approached the pituitary through a spot in the base of the skull. This was a difficult operation to master, but it allowed him to remove the pituitary without touching the brain, for when approached from this angle, the pituitary is separated from the brain above by a tough piece of tissue. Furthermore, by using this technique, Smith could be sure that the entire gland had been removed. He developed this technique to a high degree of perfection and was able to complete fifty to sixty operations a day. His mastery of this parapharyngeal approach meant that he was provided with a large number of experimental animals for the study of the pituitary. He was able to show that hypophysectomy led to the cessation of growth and the atrophy of the thyroid, adrenal cortex, and reproductive organs.[19]

Experimentation in endocrinology entailed the use of new sources of research materials. Historian Adele Clarke has described the changes in research materials necessitated by changes in methodology in the study of reproduction. In the late nineteenth and early twentieth centuries, when the morphological approach predominated, anatomists could spend a large part of their careers preparing and preserving interesting specimens. As the methods of experimental physiology began to overtake descriptive methods in the 1920s, a demand for large numbers of live animals of the same species emerged. Researchers had to develop sizable colonies of mice, rats, and guinea pigs in particular. Variations between individual animals had to be dealt with by using statistical studies of large numbers of animals and by selective breeding. Researchers hoped to develop experimental animals of such uniformity that they might be considered to be much the same as exact reagents or fine instruments.[20]

Large numbers of experimental animals were required in the work on the anterior pituitary hormones because some of these hormones acted on growth and reproduction. Such functions were not apparent in immediate and readily measurable changes in a living organism but had to be examined histologically – that is, through the microscopic study of anatomical structures. Experimental animals had to be killed at various stages of the trial, their tissues sectioned, and the shape and size of the cells of these tissue slices examined under a microscope.

Collip's work on this line of research attained particular success after 1930, when Hans Selye joined his laboratory as a research associate. Collip set him the task of learning Smith's method of hypophysectomy in the rat. Selye succeeded in mastering and further modifying the technique. Indeed, he became so proficient at it that he was able to complete the operation in five minutes while achieving an unusually low mortality rate. Within months, he was able to prepare one hundred rats per day in this way. His command of the technique provided the McGill group with the means of testing and purifying the many pituitary fractions that Collip prepared. Over the next few years, the lab members succeeded in making anterior pituitary extracts from cows, sheep, and pigs, and tested them all on Selye's hypophosectomized rats. Using this system, they were able to prepare active extracts of the thyroid-stimulating hormone and the adrenocorticotropic hormone.[21]

The combination of Collip's skills as a biochemist with those of Selye as a histologist and anatomist gave the McGill group a significant edge in pituitary research. Collip fractionated the glandular extracts while Selye provided the hypophysectomized animals and performed the histological examinations. Later, Jessie C. Williams, a registered nurse and a technician in the lab, also learned to carry out the hypophysectomies. Collip attributed his group's success to the use of large numbers of experimental animals. In one facility, for example, Collip developed an animal colony that included six to eight thousand white rats. He argued that the availability of a steady and large supply of animals was crucial to the success of their venture: "Reports in the literature on the effect of treating hypophysectomized animals with the anterior pituitary-like hormone (or 'prolan' or similar preparations) are conflicting, partly because the number of animals available for experimentation has always been small."[22]

Collip and his group set out to prepare extracts of the principles responsible for the various activities of the anterior pituitary: growth, stimulation of the thyroid, and stimulation of the adrenal cortex. The first they were able to prepare was the principle that stimulated growth in hypophysectomized rats, an activity that Evans had demonstrated many years earlier. This growth was measured in the weight gain of the animals over the course of treatment with the extract.[23]

Then, together with Evelyn Anderson, who had come from Evans's lab for post-graduate work, Collip isolated the thyroid-stimulating hormone of the pituitary, called the "thyreotropic hormone." This hormone stimulated the thyroid gland to secrete its own hormone, which in turn stimulated the body metabolism. The activity of the thyreotropic hormone could be seen in the increase in metabolism of the test animal as well as in hyperplasia of thyroid tissue. The metabolism was calculated in terms of the volume of oxygen consumed by the animal in relation to body surface and was measured in a Benedict multiple-chamber respiration apparatus. Within the thyreotropic extracts, Collip also pulled out an adrenotropic hormone that restored to normal size the atrophied adrenals in hypophysectomized rats. Histological examination of the adrenal cells showed that adrenals so treated were 50 to 300 per cent greater in weight than untreated glands. Collip and his associates are credited with priority in the preparation of extracts of the thyreotropic and adrenocorticotropic hormone (ACTH). The ACTH that Collip prepared was in a fairly crude form. Only ten years later, it was purified by two different groups: Evans and his associates Choh Hao Li and Miriam Simpson at Berkeley, and Hugh Long, Collip's former associate, and his co-workers George Sayers and Abraham White at Yale. While the adrenocorticotropic hormone was important because of its role in endocrine physiology, it took on a great therapeutic significance after 1949, when Philip Hench described the use of

cortisone in the treatment of rheumatoid arthritis. Since ACTH stimulates the release of cortisone, it began to be used therapeutically.[24]

Collip was always very protective of his children and anxious to
keep them out of harm's way. It must have been a frustrating irony for
him that at the same time he was making such progress in his hormone
research, his daughter Margaret was suffering from an endocrine disorder that he was unable to alleviate. She developed full-blown hyper-
thyroidism when she was in college and had to take complete rest.[25]

HERBERT MCLEAN EVANS

One of Collip's chief competitors in the anterior pituitary work was
Herbert McLean Evans. Evans, a leading figure in endocrinology. Evans
possessed a stellar record of achievements and a powerful, caustic personality. Collip's debates with Evans over the pituitary hormones are
remembered by Robert Noble as legendary. Evans received his bachelor
of science at Berkeley in 1904 and then trained in medicine and anatomy at Johns Hopkins for the next ten years. In 1915 he returned to
Berkeley to head the anatomy department. When he first arrived, Philip
Smith was already working on hypophysectomy, first on tadpoles and
later on rats. Evans took up the study of the pituitary, and his work in
isolating and identifying the various pituitary hormones became the focus of his research for the next forty years. He created an important
centre of research – the Institute for Experimental Biology – serving as
its director and bringing together a successful group of investigators.[26]

Victor Medvei credits Evans with being one of the first medical researchers to successfully switch from the mode of conducting research
single-handedly, or with one or two associates, to the modern pattern
of working in large teams. Evans was adept in his choice of collaborators, selecting, for example, Philip Smith and George Washington Corner. Another important fellow worker was Miriam Simpson, whose
training in medicine and chemistry complemented Evans's skill in anatomy. She used her special skills to spearhead the endocrine portion of
Evans's research program. Biochemist Choh Hao Li, also an important
associate, was a leading researcher on the chemistry of the anterior pituitary hormones. Evans and his colleague Joseph Long developed a
new strain of experimental rat – the Long-Evans rat – that was described as "attractively hooded, vigorous, but gentle, sturdy, prolific
and remarkably uniform." They established a model colony that has
been regarded as very important to the development of endocrine
research.[27]

Evans had begun his work on the anterior pituitary well over a decade before Collip. In 1920 he began working with crude extracts of

the gland, examining their ability to accelerate growth. He was able to produce giant-sized rats, and later, when he extended his experiments to other species, he created monstrous dachshunds. He and Simpson undertook a systematic effort to extract and purify the hormone responsible. The development of Smith's technique of hypophysectomy in the rat in 1926 gave impetus to Evans's study, as this new system allowed him to conduct a thorough study of the function of the various hormones. From that point through the 1930s, Evans explored many of the activities of the anterior pituitary. In 1929 he and his associates discovered that a pituitary extract stimulated the production of milk. This led other investigators to the isolation of the hormone prolactin. Two years later, Evans and Simpson identified a diabetogenic activity. In 1936 they prepared extracts of the gonadotrophic hormones and separated a follicle-stimulating hormone (FSH), luteinizing hormone (LH), and a third hormone that they called the interstitial cell-stimulating hormone (ICSH), later proved to be identical with LH.[28]

Work in this field was fiercely competitive. With so many groups working simultaneously on isolating pituitary hormones, new discoveries often occurred at approximately the same time. Worry about secrecy dogged both Evans's and Collip's groups. When Evelyn Anderson later went back to work for Evans, Collip expressed concern that she might take precious information about his extraction method to Evans. Collip, usually quite open about his work, had a particular wish to keep secrets from Evans. Abe Neufeld recalls that Collip was not very secretive and was comfortable sharing his results with almost everyone but Evans. For example, when Neufeld first arrived at the lab, he asked Collip how free he should be in discussing results with the Ayerst staff. Collip told him to treat them just the same as anybody in the department. When Neufeld gave a presentation before Rockefeller Foundation officials, Collip again told him to tell them "everything"; Neufeld thus described in detail how he developed his extracts. However, when Evans made one of his visits to Collip's lab, invariably Neufeld and the other staff would be instructed, "Don't tell him anything!" Neufeld admits, laughingly, that he "cheated on Collip once in a while." Neufeld liked Evans, and when the big, tall man came striding into the lab asking, in his booming voice, "What are you doing with those rats?" he found it difficult to hold back an honest answer.[29]

Evans, in return, complained to a Rockefeller official that Collip's group was too secretive about Selye's modifications to the hypophysectomy technique. It is not clear why Evans was irked, since the McGill group had published a detailed description of the method, one that included a precise diagram. It is interesting to note, however, that of the scores of papers produced by Collip's group during this period, all but a very few were in English, and that the key paper describing Selye's surgical method was one of these exceptions – it appeared in German in *Virchows Archiv*. This probably had more to do with German being Selye's first language than with any plot to hide information from the American competitors. Evans regularly cited scientific papers in German, so this should not have been a serious obstacle.[30]

Researchers came up with conflicting theories on the number of hormones produced by the pituitary and their precise functions. Ideas were constantly in flux. At a panel discussion on the pituitary gland in 1935, Collip was asked to comment on his current impression of the number of active fractions to be derived from pituitary tissue. He replied, "I am glad you asked me to speak as of June, 1935, because we may have quite a different impression a month or a year hence." Investigators were able to identify a growth-stimulating, a thyroid-stimulating, an adrenal cortex–stimulating, and a gonad-stimulating function. Of the gonad-stimulating fraction of the pituitary, two further functions could be identified: the stimulation of follicles and the formation of corpora lutea in the ovary. Researchers debated whether these two functions represented the action of one or two hormones. Furthermore, researchers differed on the question of whether the gonad-stimulating fraction of the pituitary was identical with the fraction isolated from pregnancy urine and the placenta, one that produced similar effects. Neither biochemical nor histological evidence alone could provide a definitive answer. While biochemical procedures could be used to isolate particular functions, it was difficult to know whether the chemical extraction process itself altered the native hormone in some way, perhaps separating segments of some master hormone molecule that carried several of these physiological functions together. Conversely, histological methods could not determine the number of active principles in a test fraction; nor did they indicate whether different principles in the fraction might be acting synergistically or antagonistically. These answers could only be attained by piecing together a puzzle by comparing extracts prepared in a variety of ways and tested systematically in different biological assay systems.[31]

Both Collip the biochemist and Evans the anatomist recognized the value of the other's skills. Collip acknowledged that the biological assays made possible by hypophysectomy had enabled his group to investigate the pituitary hormones systematically. Histological studies were important components of his group's work in preparing hormones and describing their activities. Nevertheless, when it came to finding the definitive answer, his biochemical predisposition became clear. For example, in the question of determining whether gonad-stimulating fractions of the pituitary and the placenta were identical, he said, "No one could doubt the similarity of certain physiological effects ... but the final proof of the identity of the active principle in each must be chemical."[32]

Evans, for his part, emphasized the importance of the technique of hypophysectomy. To him, these "surgical triumphs" had ushered in a new era of experimentation because the hypophysectomized rat "furnished the most conclusive test objects conceivable for replacement therapy – the only final answer as to whether or not all the essential chemical substances furnished by the gland have been captured in the extracts." However, he also clearly recognized the importance of biochemical methods. In 1933 he noted that although biological workers had been able to develop sensitive tests to give a relative assurance of the validity of distinctions made among the various pituitary substances, the ultimate demonstration that the hormones were discrete entities awaited the methods of the biochemist in concentrating and purifying the extracts. Although Evans had great respect and hopes for the contributions of biochemists in general, one might also detect his famous caustic wit at play in remarks that reveal something of his opinion of the broad sweep of Collip's endeavours: "Fortunately the biological chemist has now joined forces with the biologist or, in the example of Professor Collip, has taken charge of the whole affair, and one will sympathize with the impulse that leads me to predict that through the use of some of the most modern tools of biologic chemistry ... ultimate identification of these substances will not be long delayed."[33]

Later, in 1937, Evans continued to demonstrate a disdainful attitude towards Collip. When asked for his evaluation of Collip's group by a Rockefeller official, Evans reportedly replied that he felt Selye was gradually building up the biology of the group but that Collip was "a brilliant potshotter."[34] His attitudes perhaps reflect disciplinary jealousies and a concern that a biochemist had no business trying to do the work of the biologist as well. His "potshotter" comment, however, may have been a particularly apt critique of the overall structure of Collip's research program. Collip's intuitive and unsystematic method of making extractions and his restless urge to forge on to new territory when he felt he had finished with the most interesting part of a problem meant that while he was able to uncover much that was valuable, he often did not see things through to full fruition.

Thus, the nature of anterior pituitary hormone research forced collaboration between investigators from different disciplines. While both the biochemist and the physiologist or histologist recognized how essential the other's methods were to their research work, as individuals trained in particular disciplines, Collip and Evans tended to view the contributions from the other's discipline as valuable tools in the pursuit of their own ventures. The interdisciplinary relationship was sometimes uneasy, but for the few leading laboratories in the field, the keys to success were the mastery of the technique of hypophysectomy, the development of new supplies of research materials, and the bridging of disciplinary boundaries.

ANTIHORMONE THEORY

While working on the anterior pituitary, Collip and his co-workers were launched into a very different area of research when they followed up some anomalous observations. They found that when an animal was treated with gonadotropic hormone for a prolonged period of time, it would sometimes become resistant to the effect of the hormone. This resistance also occurred with long-term doses of thyreotropic hormone. Collip had already encountered this type of resistance in the use of parathyroid hormone in clinical treatment. This phenomenon captured his interest, and he began to carry out further research on it in 1934. He discovered that when blood serum taken from an animal that had become resistant to a particular hormone was injected into a normal animal, the second animal acquired resistance to the same substance even though it had not been exposed to the hormone before. This resistance was highly specific in that an animal that was made non-responsive to gonadotropic hormone of the pituitary would still respond to that of the placenta.

Collip argued that there were two possible explanations for this phenomenon. First, the inhibition might be due to an immunological reaction in which the injected hormone extract was the antigen and the inhibitory substance in the blood was the antibody. Alternatively, the inhibitory substance might be a normal constituent of the blood that was produced in greater amounts in response to chronic exposure to injections. He favoured the latter explanation and introduced the concept of antihormones, speculating that many or all hormones might have such an opposite – an "antihormone" – that inhibited its activity. In a healthy individual, amounts of a hormone and its antihormone would be balanced; a disease situation would occur when one of the components increased or decreased relative to the other. Collip compared the hormone-antihormone system to a buffer system in which components of the blood were carefully regulated by the balance of opposing factors. Such a theory fit with contemporary ideas of the regulation of physiological processes. The concept of buffer systems in blood chemistry was introduced by the physiologist L.J. Henderson from 1904 to 1912 and most fully elaborated during the 1920s. His ideas of a regulatory equilibrium were very influential and were extended to other bodily processes, such as temperature regulation and breathing rate, by fellow Harvard physiologist Walter B. Cannon. Cannon developed the term "homeostasis" to describe the maintenance of a dynamic equilibrium in physiological processes.[35]

A substantial portion of the work of Collip's laboratory after 1935 was devoted to the antihormone theory. Collip and Anderson prepared extracts of the sera of resistant animals and studied their antihormone properties. With Carl Bachman and Selye, he tested the resistance produced by pituitary gonadotropic hormone and APL. Among others in the field, Collip was considered "the father of antihormones." The subject was highly popular for about twenty years, becoming an area of study for laboratory researchers as well as clinicians who observed their patients develop resistance during prolonged hormone treatment.[36]

The chief criticism of this antihormone theory was that resistance might simply be an immunological response: that is, the substances attacking the hormone could be antibodies formed by the body's general defense system rather than pre-existing antihormones. While Collip acknowledged that the phenomenon he encountered "may be regarded quite rightly as a possible antibody reaction to the administered extract (antigen)," he preferred to think that the antagonistic principles were normal constituents of the blood. He was encouraged in this belief by his observation that some human patients appeared to possess antihormones to thyreotropic hormone and gonadotrophic hormone even though they had never been treated with injections. As well, histological studies indicated that the resistance extended not only to the injected hormone but also to the hormone produced by the test animal's own pituitary.[37]

HANS SELYE AND THE CONCEPT OF STRESS

Hans Selye's work began to go off in a distinctly different direction. Selye, as the youngest member of the lab, had been set the task of going to the slaughterhouse to collect buckets of cow ovaries. He was then to take the extracts that Collip made from these ovaries, inject them into female rats, and examine their sex organs for any effects. In the process, he found a number of unexpected results in the injected animals: enlarged adrenal glands, atrophied lymphatic systems, or ulcers in the stomach and upper intestine. Selye decided to experiment with extracts made from other organs as well as with toxic substances. To his surprise, these same changes occurred. He then put some of his rats on the windy roof of the building, exposing them to the Canadian winter, and others onto motorized treadmills. When both of these harsh circumstances caused the same organic changes, he postulated that in all these test cases the rats were displaying a general "alarm reaction" or the "syndrome of just being sick" rather than a reaction to any specific substance.

Gradually, Selye began to formulate his theory of the general alarm syndrome. This later became the stress theory for which he would be famous. In 1936 Selye and Collip produced a joint paper describing the interpretation of the action of various stimuli on endocrine glands; this study included a discussion of the alarm reaction produced by injections of formaldehyde. However, Selye's dogged pursuit of this line of research became a source of great friction between Collip and himself. Collip repeatedly tried to dissuade Selye from following such an uncertain course of research. In his memoirs, Selye recalled that his new idea had filled him with juvenile enthusiasm and he had been very hurt by the tough criticism of his chief, whom he respected and regarded as a fatherly friend:

When he saw me thus launched on another enraptured description of what I observed in animals treated with this or that impure toxic material, he looked at me with desperately sad eyes and cried: "But Selye, try to realize what you are doing before it is too late! You have now decided to spend your entire life studying the meaningless side effects of disease. I am even tempted to look upon your work as the pharmacology of dirt!"[38]

Eventually, the dispute between the two men became insupportable. Selye left the department in 1938 and, fortunately, was able to find a new home in the anatomy department. This regrettable rift was due to both personal and intellectual factors. On the personal level, it was a clash of two strong-minded individuals. Selye was noted for his arrogance. His strong commitment to a project that Collip found valueless was incompatible with the system that Collip had established in his laboratory. Although lab members were permitted a great deal of freedom in pursuing their interests, it was always Collip who set the broader questions and themes that they were to follow. Selye's theory was out of step with Collip's research program on an intellectual level: Selye was concerned with a general, widespread, non-specific response, while Collip's work was devoted to specificity. Collip focused on identifying distinct activities, extracting and purifying the principles responsible for them, and then precisely defining their chemical and physiological properties.[39]

In his concept of the alarm reaction, Selye took a very different approach to explaining resistance (or at least certain instances of resistance) than Collip had with his antihormone theory. Selye explored situations in which hormone resistance developed but no antihormone substance could be demonstrated in the blood. He found that this resistance was not very specific. An animal rendered resistant through treatment with estradiol, for example, was also resistant to the synthetic estrogen diethylstilbestrol. He interpreted this as evidence that the animal had developed a resistance not to the chemical substance itself but to the toxic effect of the principle and that this resistance followed the pattern of general adaptation to any noxious stimulus. He gradually developed a theory of the general adaptation syndrome, which he described as "the sum of all non-specific, systemic reactions of the body which ensue upon long continued exposure to stress" and which are distinct from specific adaptive reactions such as the development of muscles upon physical exercise or allergic and immunological reactions to foreign agents.[40]

Collip was committed to his antihormone theory but was careful to maintain that it was a working hypothesis. In 1938 he acknowledged that true antibodies were doubtless formed and that the question of whether antihormones were also present could only be decided after much more experimental work. In his final article on the subject in 1941, Collip, with Selye and Thomson, discussed the large body of literature that had provided evidence both for and against the antihormone theory. One of the issues emphasized in the article was the importance of the factor of species specificity. Three different animals from three different species could be involved in such experiments: the animal from which the original extract was taken, the one into which the extract was injected, and the final animal that received the serum of the second.[41]

Herbert Evans was highly sceptical about the existence of antihormones, especially because his own studies with growth hormone had shown that as the hormone preparations were purified, they were less likely to cause the type of response associated with antihormones. During a discussion of a paper about antihormone therapy at the 1948 Laurentian Hormone Conference, Evans offered these sarcastic remarks:

No more brilliant observation has ever been made in the history of experimental biology than that of Collip and Anderson who observed that animals treated chronically with such anterior hypophyseal preparations as were then available failed to provide continuous physiological stimulation although their extracts were active in fresh animals. My cheeks, however, are lined with creases to the depth of the Grand Canyon as our colleagues employed the term "antihormone" for the phenomenon of refractoriness and they will be credited forever in the world's history of accurate knowledge for this term. A refractory phase will almost inevitably ensue with impure preparations but will disappear, will melt like ice in the sun, with purification of the material in question.[42]

Later, endocrine scientist Roy Greep suggested that the idea of anti-hormones "caught the fancy of researchers and mushroomed ... this ideological balloon did not burst when punctured by fact but deflated ever so slowly during the next fifteen years." As opposing evidence built up, the idea of antihormones gradually lost out to the theory that resistance was due to an immunological reaction. Robert Noble and David Thomson rationalized, however, that one legacy of the antihor-mone theory was that it successfully raised the question of species spec-ificity in the use of protein hormones in therapeutic procedures.[43]

ONGOING STUDIES
OF THE PARATHYROID HORMONE

The study of the parathyroid hormone and its physiological activities continued to interest Collip. He and his associates made significant contributions to the understanding of the manner in which this hor-mone acted. Theodore Schwartz provides an account of a friendly intel-lectual contest between Collip and Fuller Albright in the mid-1930s and early 1940s over the question of how the hormone acted to control calcium metabolism. Collip argued that the hormone acted on the bone, while Albright argued that it acted on the kidneys. This contest continued for some time, up until 1942 when, after performing an ex-periment, Collip and Abe Neufeld were forced to admit that Albright was correct in saying the hormone acted on the kidneys. Albright agreed with the conclusion but disagreed that Collip's experiment had proven the point. Ironically, some time later, Albright turned around and conceded that the hormone acted on the bone. Schwartz calls Collip and Albright "giants with tunnel vision" because they insisted on a single action for the hormone. He attributes this tendency to the "intuitive parsimonious appeal" of the idea that a hormone would act on only one target organ, in analogy to the action of insulin on blood glucose. Albright's associate Read Ellsworth, not emotionally bound to either stance, finally recognized that the two positions were un-necessarily polarized, that in fact the parathyroid hormone acted at both sites.[44]

Albright also expressed interest in Collip's idea of antihormones and wrote to Collip when he began encountering resistance to parathyroid hormone in a patient who had never received parathyroid treatment before. In his reply, Collip suggested a method for testing antiparathy-roid substance in the serum of the patient. Albright later rejected the antihormone explanation for this phenomenon and developed the theory of end-organ resistance for pseudohypoparathyroidism. This theory held that while many of the symptoms of this condition were like those of normal hypoparathyroidism, the patients failed to react to parathyroid injections, not because of acquired resistance but because their receptor organs were constitutionally unable to respond. Christiane Sinding has examined the development of Albright's theory and his rejection of Collip's idea of antihormones.[45]

Collip's great years began to ebb towards the end of the decade. David Thomson's teaching responsibilities grew ever larger. Evelyn Anderson returned to Berkeley. The nature of the department's experimental work changed after Selye's departure in 1938 even though Selye continued to help with histological reports. Greater emphasis was put on studying those pituitary factors that caused changes that could be evaluated through physiological measurements such as oxygen consumption and blood sugar level rather than those that required histological study. For example, Collip and Abe Neufeld studied the effects of pituitary extracts on fat and carbohydrate metabolism.

Collip continued to work with a large group of students and associates, and together they explored a wide variety of topics, such as the prolactin and diabetogenic activities of the anterior pituitary and the effects of testosterone, adrenaline, and estrin. One less successful venture was a pituitary extract that Collip named "No. 622" after his family's new home on 622 Sydenham Avenue in Westmount. With Abe Neufeld and Orville Denstedt, he studied its effect in stimulating metabolism. When volunteers in the lab took it by oral administration, they reported that it gave rise to feelings of vigour and well-being. With I.M. Rabinowitch at the Montreal General Hospital, Collip and his co-workers conducted clinical trials of "622" in the hope that it might have uses in the treatment of obesity or in cases where an increase in metabolism was desirable. The existence of this substance was never clearly demonstrated, however, and clinical trials failed to reveal any activity that could be attributed to it.[46]

THE WAR

Upon Canada's entrance into the Second World War in 1939, many medical researchers across the country began to direct their research activities to supporting the war effort. Collip and his lab were no exception. With Robert Noble, Collip examined the problem of shock and the production of mammary tumours upon treatment with diethylstilbestrol and other forms of estrogen. The research on shock was of particular importance in wartime. Noble and Collip experimented with a number of ways of producing trauma in rats, such as crushing or freezing their extremities. They finally developed a revolving upright circular drum (known as the Noble-Collip drum) in which they spun rats. The rats were traumatized, carried upward and then dropped as the drum turned, but did not suffer obvious hemorrhages or fractures. The amount of trauma could be quantified by regulating the time the rats were subjected to the treatment. The Noble-Collip drum was picked up by other researchers but caused outrage among antivivisectionists.[47]

After 1941 Collip's research productivity dropped off dramatically. He became increasingly involved in wartime administrative work with the medical research arm of the National Research Council and had to spend much of his time travelling between Montreal, Ottawa, and Washington. During the years he was away from the laboratory, he was increasingly left behind by the continued advances in knowledge and laboratory technique.

His old rival, Herbert Evans, along with Choh Hao Li and Miriam Simpson achieved some of the most important successes during this period: a purified ACTH in 1943, growth hormone in 1944, and follicle-stimulating hormone (FSH) in 1949. Evans continued to collaborate successfully with skilled biochemists. In reference to the isolation of the adrenocorticotrophic hormone, he said, "In order to establish the biological characteristic of a hormone from a complex source such as the pituitary, it must first be isolated in pure form judged both by *chemical* and *biological* data." He emphasized the importance of the interplay of chemical and biological methods in the purification of growth hormone. One of the keys to the success of Evans and his collaborators was the development of a very sensitive bioassay that involved examining the thickness of the epiphysial plate of the tibia of young hypophysectomized rats, a tissue that was very responsive to growth hormone.[48] Despite the rift with Selye, Collip and Thomson continued to write review papers with him and to ask for his services in making histological examinations. Selye, however, was becoming more and more occupied with his general adaptation theory. Without Selye as a member of his team, Collip did not have ready access to the innovative work in anatomy and histology that the Evans group used to great effect.

Another factor in the decline of Collip's work was the advent of new techniques in biochemistry. His colleague Robert Noble explained that during the war Collip's field of protein extraction changed dramatically. "His familiar techniques had given way to strange technical and mechanical methods of separation, enabling isolation, identification and even synthesis of polypeptide chains."[49] Among these new techniques were electrophoresis and ultracentrifugation, both of which were used by the groups led by Evans at Berkeley and Hugh Long at Yale in 1943 in isolating ACTH. These methods utilized physical properties of the component molecules to separate them mechanically and to demonstrate that the final products were homogeneous. They allowed Evans and Long to go beyond the crude extract of adrenocorticotropic hormone that Collip and Anderson had prepared in 1933.

The equipment used by the Berkeley and Yale researchers was not readily available to Canadians until some time later. The electrophoresis technique was introduced by Arne Wilhelm Kaurin Tiselius of the University of Uppsala in 1937. The first electrophoresis instruments in Canada were installed at Dalhousie and Alberta about 1948 and at the National Research Council in 1950. The ultracentrifuge had been developed by Svedberg in 1924, but few actual examples of it existed for many years after, as it was a huge machine, driven by an oil turbine and requiring two floors of space. A more compact, analytical ultracentrifuge was first installed in Canada in 1949 at the National Research Council at the cost of $20,000.[50] Collip did not use any of these methods in his scientific work, perhaps because he did not have ready access to the equipment. Since Collip was, by that date, head of the National Research Council Medical Research Committee (later Division), it seems likely that he could have availed himself of the opportunity had he felt it important. More likely, his administrative work had taken him away from the bench for so long that he chose not to tackle learning these new methods, recognizing how difficult it would be for him to return to the forefront of research.

EVERYTHING WAS GOOD FUN

The hectic decade of the 1930s saw the peak of Collip's research career. He had been the head of a large, thriving laboratory group and on the cutting edge of one of the most exciting fields of research. He was later to look back upon this period with a fondness rivalling that for his insulin days. In 1964 Herbert Evans asked him to prepare a statement for a publication on the endocrines, asking him to recall what researches had given him the most fun. Collip replied:

As far as "fun" is concerned, that on a certain time in January 1922 at about midnight when I found that I could trap insulin in 80%–95% alcohol I nearly went crazy with joy! ... Naturally, as you have guessed, I got a great kick out of my work on the parathyroid (1924–26) and of the pituitary work at McGill in the 30's. I think I would have to put ACTH first although for about 10 years everything was good fun.[51]

He had achieved this productivity by successfully making the transition from working as an individual to heading a large team of investigators. Moreover, the team was particularly successful when it was anchored by the ideal configuration of Collip and Selye with their complementary skills in biochemistry and histology. Collip was most happy at the centre of his laboratory, fractionating a continuous stream of hormones that his associates were set to test.

Collip's problems arose when this pattern of activity broke down. He gave his co-workers a great deal of freedom in determining their projects; in fact, his critics have suggested that Collip's group was too ambitious in pursuing a broad range of topics and not sufficiently thorough in following them through, that they tried to cover too much ground in too little time.[52] Collip, however, could not brook the extreme challenge posed by Selye to his research program. Selye's subsequent departure was a grave loss to Collip's work.

While Collip made important contributions to physiological theory, such as his conclusions about the mechanism of the action of the parathyroid hormone, his most significant achievements were in manipulative biochemistry rather than in theory. He was at his best when pulling out thyreotrophic hormone and adrenotrophic hormone, as he had been with insulin and parathyroid hormone. He was less successful when he ventured into the conceptual realm, as with the antihormone theory. Beginning in the 1940s, the field of protein chemistry began to change dramatically. The new instruments and methods were a far cry from those used in Collip's intuitive, "bathtub" style of chemistry. The methods that had brought him so much success for decades were now being overtaken by the techniques developed by a new generation.

6

The Private Funding
of Research, 1928–1947:
Patents, Grants, and Institutes

I do not wish to enlarge my staff to any appreciable extent, but I should like to
be able to keep my workers together.[1]

J.B. Collip to C.F. Martin, 15 December 1934

Scientific knowledge is a product not only of experiments and ideas but
also of institutions and financial resources. During the period he was at
McGill, Collip had a distinct vision for his research enterprise and was
continually engaged in negotiations with parties both inside and outside the university to make this dream a reality. In the mid- to late
1930s, one of Collip's prime concerns was to ensure the financial stability of his laboratory group. To this end, he and Charles Martin made
a bid to the Rockefeller Foundation for a research grant. Collip was
also engaged in a series of discussions with McGill University officials
to further his goal of gaining greater status, stability, and the freedom
to concentrate on his research.

During the 1930s, there was no large-scale, systematic governmental
funding of medical research in Canada. The National Research Council
of Canada (NRC) directed fellowships and grants only towards work in
the physical sciences. A notable exception to this pattern was the NRC
support of tuberculosis research during the 1920s and 1930s. Experimental work in the medical sciences was largely carried out in academic
settings; there, research work was supported primarily by general university funds provided by the provincial governments. McGill and the University of Toronto were the leading universities in the country and the
only two institutions to offer fully developed doctoral programs until after the Second World War. McGill differed from Toronto in that it derived the bulk of its funding from private sources. Because of this,
McGill was much more dependent upon the bounty of the business community, wealthy alumni, and philanthropic foundations, particularly the

Rockefeller Foundation and the Carnegie Foundation. The Banting Research Foundation, established in 1925 as a legacy of the insulin discovery, was one of the few Canadian sources of medical research funds.[2]

From the mid-1930s to the early 1940s, the McGill administration underwent a period of instability, running through a rapid succession of principals. Sir Arthur Currie, the university's hero-principal, died of pneumonia in November of 1933. McGill's chancellor, Edward Wentworth Beatty, took over as acting principal for over a year, until a successor was named in June 1935. Beatty, past president of the Canadian Pacific Railway, had been a strong and active chancellor. He had been a dominant figure at the university even during Currie's term as principal, and especially during Currie's extended absences, illness, and in the final years of his life. After Currie's death, Beatty exercised what McGill historian Stanley Frost calls "his own brand of benevolent dictatorship" until the end of the decade.[3]

After the First World War, McGill's Faculty of Medicine was systematically revitalized and its research facilities expanded. The medical institutions created out of this reform were strongly oriented towards scientific research and to the close association of basic science and clinical science. One of the most notable developments was the establishment of the University Medical Clinic in conjunction with the Royal Victoria Hospital in 1924. Jonathan Meakins's great achievement there was to bring the basic sciences and the spirit of scientific inquiry to clinical medicine. The clinic became home to an active group of researchers in the basic and clinical sciences. The Montreal Neurological Institute was another notable institution created around this time. When Wilder Penfield, the renowned neurosurgeon, was invited to McGill in 1928 as professor of neurology and neurosurgery, he proposed the establishment of an institute that would serve as a clinical hospital and a research facility. Such an institute was completed in 1934, built with the aid of $1,282,652 from the Rockefeller Foundation, $400,000 from the Quebec government, $300,000 from the City of Montreal, and $125,000 from various research funds within the university. The Montreal Neurological Institute gained an international reputation for its achievement in research and treatment. The third accomplishment was the creation of the Pathological Institute in 1924, in collaboration with the Royal Victoria Hospital and under the direction of Horst Oertel. This institute housed the McGill pathology and bacteriology departments, provided pathological and bacteriological services to the hospital, and served as a centre of clinical studies.[4]

In appointing Collip, Martin was adding another distinguished medical scientist to his faculty and thus furthering McGill's research reputation. Collip proved his worth by greatly expanding the research program of the Department of Biochemistry. As we have seen, through the 1930s, he headed a large and energetic group of investigators who produced a remarkable stream of papers in endocrinology. Warren Weaver of the Rockefeller Foundation observed, "Members of this Department constitute a very unusual group in intelligence, enthusiasm and loyalty to their chief. Investigators come here from Canada, the States, and England, and apparently they all want to stay on indefinitely."[5] The size and energy of Collip's group were a credit to his skill as a leader and a scientist, but the responsibility of supporting a large number of staff proved to be a heavy burden.

When Collip first arrived at McGill in 1928, the departmental budget was $21,000. In just six years, he managed to more than double that figure to $51,500. A large portion of the budget came from general university funds, but cutbacks in university finances since the start of the Depression had reduced this amount from $26,000 to $18,000 (or from over half of the total departmental expenditures to just one-third). Collip was obliged to raise the remainder of the departmental funds from outside sources. For Collip, the most significant source of research funds throughout his career was the insulin royalties. As beneficiaries of the insulin royalties, he, Banting, and Best shared in what Michael Bliss argues was "probably the largest pool of Canadian capital supporting medical research" until the Second World War, a fact that put these three in financial positions rivalled by few other medical scientists in the country. From 1930 to 1935, Collip's portion of the royalties increased steadily from $20,000 to $30,000 per annum. At McGill, only the University Clinic and the Neurological Institute had the same degree of stable funding: the University Clinic endowment provided an annual income of $24,000 and the Neurological Institute endowment yielded $40,000.[6]

In later years, Collip also collected royalties from the other products he developed. Emmenin royalties amounted to only one or two thousand dollars annually in the first few years of its commercial life, but once Ayerst moved into the American market, sales jumped dramatically. By 1939 McGill was receiving $22,000 a year. Sales of Emmenin dropped after 1940 owing to competition from synthetic forms of estrogen, but Ayerst then developed the highly successful Premarin, a natural estrogen that, like Emmenin, was orally active. Ayerst advertised Collip's name on its labels and used the services of his laboratory for the standardization of this new product. Although Collip had not been directly involved in the development of Premarin, Ayerst paid him a 2 per cent royalty, perhaps in recognition of the credibility the product gained through its association with his name and perhaps in gratitude for the success his collaboration had brought them. This proved to be no small token. By

1947 Premarin royalties brought in over $50,000 per year. Royalties from Pituitrin, also produced by Ayerst, provided another few thousand dollars a year. Collip, concerned for the long-term stability of his finances, had the funds from these royalties capitalized in order to build up a substantial endowment.[7]

Short-term grants from individual benefactors had a less significant place in the departmental budget. These donations were usually made only for a period of one or two years, providing an additional $5,000 to $10,000 for research. They offered none of the security of the other sources of income and were dependent upon Collip's skill in cultivating the friendship and support of such leading Canadian philanthropists as Vincent Massey and Samuel Bronfman.[8]

Vincent Massey was the grandson of Hart Massey, founder of Massey-Harris, the leading manufacturer of agricultural machinery. As chairman of the Massey Foundation, created out of Hart's estate, Vincent effectively controlled the many large benefactions made by the foundation. Massey's younger son, Hart, had had an operation at the age of six that had affected his pituitary gland; the result was that at the age of sixteen, he remained very small. Massey consulted a wide group of medical experts, including Collip and Selye, about his son's endocrine problem. The famous neurosurgeon Harvey Cushing operated on Hart as well. Very impressed by what they had heard of Collip's research work and by what they had seen in his laboratories, Massey and his wife made several annual grants of $5,000 from the Massey Foundation to Collip's work starting in 1933.[9]

THE ROCKEFELLER FOUNDATION BID

The funding collected from these various sources was sufficient to carry Collip's department through its most active phase of research in the 1930s. By mid-decade, however, a number of concerns began to weigh heavily on Collip. First, the physical facilities for his team's work were stretched to the limit. The biochemistry department was located with the other biological science departments in the new Biological Building that had been completed with Rockefeller money in 1922. When it was first constructed, the building had been a celebrated example of the latest in laboratory design, but by the mid-1930s the laboratory space and animal-care facilities proved inadequate for Collip's rapidly expanding research group. Second, Collip faced the probable loss of his insulin royalties. The insulin patents, the single largest source of his research monies, were due to expire in 1940. In his desire to ensure the continuation of the work of his group beyond the 1940 deadline, Collip turned to the Rockefeller Foundation, which had so handsomely endowed the

Neurological Institute and many other medical facilities at McGill. His vision for his research group is revealed in his application to the foundation.

During the 1920s, the Rockefeller Foundation made a series of large grants to the building program of McGill's medical faculty. From 1925 to 1928, the foundation's administrative structure underwent a major reorganization that produced a significant change in its granting policy. The foundation's various divisions were realigned in order to consolidate their activities and to rein in some of the more powerful boards. The restructuring shifted the foundation's focus from medicine and public health, which had been its traditional areas of strength, towards a greater emphasis on science. Five divisions were created: the International Health Division, which was responsible for public health, and divisions for natural sciences, medical sciences, social sciences, and humanities. Because the Great Depression made large and long-term projects too expensive, the foundation changed its emphasis from large grants for institution building to small, short-term grants for individual projects and to systematic support for work in specific fields designated by foundation officers. This new system was carried out by professional philanthropic staff members who have been described by historian Robert Kohler as "activist programme managers." These officers were sufficiently well versed in their fields to select particular lines of research for concentration and to make judgments about individual applications. In December 1933 Warren Weaver, head of the foundation's natural sciences division, and Alan Gregg, head of the medical sciences division, formulated a joint program called "psychobiology." Psychobiology encompassed psychiatry and the sciences underlying human behaviour. In addition to psychiatry, psychology, and neurophysiology, this program included the sub-fields of nutrition, radiation, sex physiology, embryology, genetics, general physiology, biophysics and biochemistry, and internal secretions. Weaver was responsible for basic research in each of these areas, and Gregg looked after the clinical portion.[10]

Collip had had his first contact with the Rockefeller Foundation when he had received his travelling fellowship 1921. It was during the term of this award that he had travelled to Toronto and had embarked on the work on insulin. As early as 1929, Collip's program at McGill was being considered for research aid by the officers of the foundation. Collip was well thought of by a number of Rockefeller managers. R.M. Pearce, then head of the medical sciences division, remarked in 1929, "Collip is an excellent man ... He is really a biochemist, and one of the best ... and I may add that as a result of my first contact with him nine years ago when he was at the University of Alberta, he received one of our fellowships."[11]

In 1934 Collip and Martin began to formulate a bid to the natural sciences division headed by Warren Weaver. The frank entries that Weaver and other foundation officers made in their diaries reveal their perceptions of Collip's application. Weaver first visited Collip at McGill in February 1934, and in his report to his assistant director, Frank Blair Hanson, he expressed his approval of what he saw of Collip and his staff. Hanson noted: "WW [Weaver] is very favourably impressed by C. [Collip] by the program of his group, and by the intelligence and industry of all the staff. C. has collected and attracted a really remarkable crowd of young people, all of whom seem quite on fire with enthusiasm. The laboratory is going full steam from early morning until midnight and later."[12]

During Weaver's meeting with Collip, Collip explained to him that his ultimate objective was the creation of an institute of endocrinology, either in a separate building or in the Biological Building, where he was then located. He suggested that this had been one of the plans that Sir Arthur Currie had hoped to put into effect before his death in 1933. Collip was most intensely concerned however, about difficulties maintaining the financial support of his group; there was so little stability in his budget, he noted, and he did not wish to spend so much of his own time soliciting funds year by year. Weaver was impressed that Collip did not have any grandiose ideas for expansion, noting that Collip had said he would be exceedingly happy just to have his situation stabilized at or near its existing level. Collip's idea of establishing a separate institute derived from his long-cherished wish to devote himself entirely to his research work, away from the teaching and administrative responsibilities entailed in chairing a university department. Only a few models for this type of institute existed in Canada, the most significant being the Banting and Best Department of Medical Research at the University of Toronto, which had grown out of a research chair created for Frederick Banting in 1923. McGill's Neurological Institute and Pathological Institute, a short distance up Mount Royal from Collip's home in the Biological Building, were other examples of research institutes, but in these places, original research was closely associated with clinical treatment.[13]

Since Weaver was a mathematical physicist, he sought the advice of others when it came to matters relating to biomedical science. Soon after his visit to Montreal, he consulted with two of Collip's peers in the field, both of them active in the study of anterior pituitary hormones – Philip Smith at Berkeley and Earl Theron Engle at Columbia. While Smith and Engle told Weaver that they recognized that Collip was a very important investigator, Weaver noted in his diary their comments to the effect that Collip had "tried to cover too much ground and that his work has been somewhat too hurried." This criticism was later shared by others, and it proved to be of key importance in determining the fate of the grant application.[14]

Martin and Collip were very stimulated by Weaver's visit and asked for a further interview with him at his office the following month when they were to be in New York for a conference and lectures. At that meeting, Weaver, Martin, and Collip discussed in general terms the levels at which the foundation might consider supporting Collip's work. At the lowest level of commitment, the foundation could simply provide assistance for individual projects. More generously, the foundation might provide some help to stabilize the departmental budget. At a higher level yet, the foundation might provide both budget stabilization and some funds for basic equipment. Finally, and ideally, the Rockefeller Foundation could construct and endow new quarters for the group, consisting of a new wing to the building or perhaps a small building for the institute. They agreed that no plans would go further until the fall, when the university would have developed a more definite plan with financial estimates.[15]

In December of 1934 Martin returned to New York and submitted a more detailed application. This time he met with Alan Gregg, the head of the medical sciences division, to discuss the clinical aspects of the work. Weaver, laid up in the hospital for six weeks, was unable to meet with him. Martin brought along a memorandum in which Collip articulated his dreams for his group:

It is my wish that my department should develop into an endocrine research institute. Endocrinology is an exceedingly broad and comprehensive subject, and in order that it may advance as a whole, it follows that advances must be made simultaneously in many of its various subdivisions. Probably nowhere else in the world is there a more advantageous setting for endocrine research than here at McGill, with the department of Biochemistry as the nucleus. Here, under one roof ... divergent phases of the subject are being studied.[16]

Perhaps aware of the criticisms made against his broadly based program, Collip added: "The ... list of our activities may at first sight suggest that we are undertaking too ambitious a program. My answer to such criticism would be simply this: that we have been carrying on in this way for a number of years and all we ask is that we be allowed to continue in our work." Again, Collip emphasized that his main concern was for stability rather than for expansion.

I do not wish to enlarge my staff to any appreciable extent, but I should like *to be able to keep my workers together*. This will involve a much greater salary budget for the future. Our working quarters are far from adequate, and they should be at least doubled. The present staff could make use of more space and equipment and the output of work would be increased. We are particularly badly off as regards the proper housing, etc. of our experimental animals, and certain very important types of work which we are otherwise fully equipped to do cannot be done on account of this.[17]

He emphasized his department's favourable situation, specifically its friendly relations with various hospitals so that he and his group could learn of endocrine cases of special interest. Perhaps playing to Weaver's interest in supporting investigations related to human behaviour, Collip added that he felt there was particular opportunity for applying laboratory studies to psychiatric cases and behavioural problems. He added that the department was organized so that "there is continual dovetailing and interlacing of all the experimental work" thanks to the relationship the individual workers had with him and to various lateral working arrangements he established from time to time.[18]

Upon returning to Montreal, Martin wrote Gregg asking him to visit Montreal to see the clinical end of the work as well as the Neurological Institute that Gregg's division had been responsible for building. When this invitation was not accepted, Collip and Martin made a return visit to New York in March 1935 to see Weaver and Gregg. This time they were accompanied by Hector Mortimer, a physician who was working in Collip's laboratory on a voluntary basis. Collip had hoped to provide Mortimer with some support for his studies. This member of the party proved not to be an asset, however. Warren Weaver reported on the meeting in his diary: "An unfortunate proportion of the available time taken up by Mortimer's elaborate and somewhat glib presentation of his conception of the field of endocrinology and its applications. It is not clear whether Mortimer is present as a chosen and effective spokesman or because, out of concern for his own future, he may have insisted upon his inclusion."[19]

Following Mortimer's presentation, Martin broached the subject of the funds that were being requested, suggesting that approximately $200,000 would be required to remodel, modernize, and fireproof the old portion of the Biological Building for the use of Collip's department. Gregg made it clear that such a sum was not likely to be forthcoming at that time. Weaver noted of the discussion: "Somewhat vague presentation of requirements for the research program in endocrinology, the vagueness apparently having its origin in the fact that Martin would like to ask for as much as there is any possible chance of his getting and therefore does not wish to expose his hand until the Foundation shall have given him some indication. Lacking this indication, the information is not very definite or satisfactory."[20]

Indeed, two subjects appear to have been up for discussion: first, the request for support for the research program that was in place, with some possible additions, and second, the issue of how to replace the income derived from the insulin patents. Weaver again noted the vagueness of the McGill delegation in this latter matter: "The group appears not to know just when this insulin income will cease through expiration of the patents." His general sense after the meeting was that only interim assistance could be considered for the time being and that this would be for the most pressing needs, such as space for animals. He noted in conclusion: "The interview is not a very satisfactory one. Collip, the substantial member of the group, gets relatively little opportunity to express his ideas." Alan Gregg added in his own diary, "I am dubious as to the credibility of Mortimer but Collip's work is important and deserves some sort of aid."[21]

In order to gain a better sense of the potential costs involved in creating additional space in the Biological Building, Martin asked the superintendent engineer at McGill to draw up an estimate. The existing building was in the shape of an "I," the northern wing of which was the portion of the old medical building that had been spared from the fire of 1907. The central and southern portions of the building were the sections built in 1922. The biochemistry department, which occupied the third floor of the new section, had offices, research and teaching laboratories, a library, and storerooms. The engineering report made it clear that it was not feasible to reconstruct the old part of the Biological Building, and proposed instead various schemes to add a new storey over the existing building, the estimates for which ranged from $19,000 to $73,000. These plans included new rooms and accommodations for the rat colony and the monkeys.[22]

Hoping that the application could be considered by the foundation trustees at their spring meeting, Martin wrote to Weaver to follow up on their most recent interview. He argued: "Professor Collip and his associates have already made a number of outstanding contributions, and his recent discoveries, which seem most important of all, give promise of greater achievement. He is at the most productive period of his life, and should be vigorous and active for at least fifteen to twenty years. This is the time he most of all needs every possible facility."[23]

This time, Martin considerably scaled down the ambitious figure of $200,000 that he had suggested at the earlier meeting. He proposed an alternative construction scheme that could be carried out for $60,000, and suggested that it should satisfy Collip's needs for many years to come. Martin asked that the foundation provide $40,000 of this sum and offered to raise the rest of the amount from other sources. In addition, he asked for an annual sum of $20,000 for four years for personnel and supplies. This sum was not to be used to provide any additional appointments to the staff, but only to help pay for technical assistance, apparatus, supplies, and animals. Collip argued that this amount would simply allow his existing staff to work at maximum efficiency and that it would increase their productivity considerably. Martin acknowledged the fact that the insulin royalties were due to expire soon but insisted that Collip would carry on his work after that, even on a skeleton budget if he had to. "On the other hand," he ventured, "we feel that by that time his results will be such as to stimulate further interest in his work both at home and abroad."[24]

In New York, Weaver was not impressed by this presentation; he found it lacking in that it did not contain an explicit statement of the department's financial situation. In his diary, he noted that "it seemed clear that Martin should be able, and be required, to indicate in full detail the sources of present and future income for support of Collip's work. In the absence of an entirely clear picture of this phase of things, I see no reason for aid from RF." In a reply to Martin, Weaver asked for further details of the budget of the department – where the income came from and what proportion of it the foundation money was to replace, details of plans, and estimates for remodelling – "so that it is clear that $60,000 will accomplish a result which is really satisfactory from the scientific point of view." Most critically, he asked, "Is it wise to expand considerably with the knowledge that the insulin income will decrease or drop out in 1939?" He dashed Martin's hope that the application would be considered that spring and indicated that it could not be reviewed until the fall.[25]

This came as a blow to Collip and Martin. Collip commented to a friend and former colleague, University of Alberta zoologist William Rowan, "I have had rather a serious disappointment in regard to securing extra money for expanding the work. I hope that this is only a temporary setback, but in these day one cannot be sure of anything unless he has the money in hand."[26]

At the end of August, Martin tried again. He wrote to Weaver saying that he and Collip were very anxious to have another opportunity to discuss the matter. He added that work had been going well during the summer and "some very interesting new light has been thrown on a number of new problems." Another meeting was arranged, but it, too, failed to achieve the desired outcome. Weaver wrote in his diary afterwards that before Collip's arrival Martin had made "a characteristically silly inquiry as to whether he has 'offended' some officer of the

Foundation, his sensitivity apparently arising from the fact that we are not rushing through his requests on his own schedule." Martin tried to impress on Weaver the poor financial situation at McGill. The university had been running a $250,000 deficit and, by strenuous measures, had reduced this to about $100,000. Martin mentioned a recent large bequest to the medical school (he was perhaps referring to one from the William G. Cheney estate) that had already produced $50,000 and was expected to produce some $30,000 or $35,000 more for work in medicine. Martin had hoped to use a fair portion of this money for Collip's building program, but the Board of Governors had decided to use only the income and not touch the principal. When Weaver inquired about whether other funds from private sources might be anticipated, he noted that neither Martin nor Collip appeared to welcome the question and that "both are a little vague in their general indication that no further money is in sight."[27]

In terms of detailed financial information, the McGill delegation came to this meeting better prepared than before. Martin presented Weaver with an official statement of the income and expenditures for the department for the year 1934–35, along with five sheets showing the details of the salaries and wages of the staff. Weaver, scrupulous in his observations, quickly noted that the totals for the salaries did not match on the two different statements. Collip tried to remedy the gaff by explaining that the accounting process by which the salaries were assigned to the various sources of income was a wholly artificial process. He went through the list of salaries, quickly marking T's and P's next to the names of those he considered to be temporary or permanent members of the staff. Trying to regain his footing, Collip moved the discussion on to the larger question of his two main goals. The first was to give his present staff satisfactory accommodation. The second was to replace the income then gained from one-time private donations – about $10,000 – and, after July 1940, to replace the income from the insulin royalties. Collip stated dramatically that if he could not obtain some pledge of outside assistance for the years after 1940, he would immediately begin to cut his staff and accumulate a reserve from the insulin income.[28]

When the pair returned to Montreal, Martin quickly tried to further repair their blunder by sending corrected salary figures to Weaver with an explanation of the discrepancy between the two sets of figures they had presented. This was to no avail. Ten days after the interview, Weaver responded with a clear "no." He explained that the foundation was unwilling to contribute the funds requested to maintain a level of expenditure that would only have to be reduced when the insulin patents ended. He emphasized that he was not prejudging whether or not the foundation would be willing to replace the insulin income after 1940 but only that it was impossible for him to make such a pledge at that time. He suggested grimly that they would be well advised to reduce the budget of the department. He concluded, "It therefore seems to me that this is an inappropriate moment to consider support of the budget of the department." He offered only this: "Were the University in a position to assure the replacement of the insulin income, the situation would obviously be greatly altered." As for the matter of the building program, again he was negative. He explained that revised foundation policies now inclined against expenditures for "brick and mortar." "It seems clear to me that I could not possibly hope for a favorable reaction to a proposal that the Foundation furnish all of the sum required for the proposed rebuilding. If the University can obtain from internal or other sources a fair fraction of the necessary amount, we are prepared, as in all other cases, to study the proposal. It goes without saying that the probability for a favorable decision would increase, the larger the amount that can be furnished by the University." Martin wrote back to express his disappointment with the result but stated his intention to take the matter up with the new principal and to renew his bid at a later date.[29]

The only further contact that Collip had with foundation officials that year was in October when Harry Miller, assistant director of the natural sciences division, made a surprise visit to Collip's laboratory. Collip talked to him about his antihormone theory and gave him a rapid tour of the department. Miller was impressed that although he had arrived unannounced, "almost all the staff were present, and the place was a beehive of activity." Collip and Miller had some discussion of the financial state of the department. Collip explained that Martin had no assurance of local support for the building program but was sure that some would certainly be found if the foundation were to award a grant. Although Miller professed to know nothing about such a possibility, he gently suggested that he had his doubts whether the foundation would get involved in such a situation, knowing that it would change in a matter of a few years and that a large annual sum would be necessary to maintain the existing level of research. Miller noted in his diary that in spite of the uncertainties of the financial situation and the threat to the quality of animal material because of overcrowded animal quarters, Collip was planning an expansion of his research program.[30]

In June 1935 McGill named its new principal. Arthur Morgan arrived from England, where he had gained a name in the administration of Hull College. Stanley Frost explained that the chancellor, Beatty, and the new principal took an instant dislike to each other. They had diver-

gent views on a number of important questions, including their politics; whereas the chancellor was politically conservative, the principal
was "a little inclined to the left."[31] This may have had only a little
to do with Morgan's problems, though. Frost remarked, "Any new
principal coming into office was going to find it difficult to discover
his own position of authority," since Beatty, his associate George
McDonald, a governor and chairman of the finance committee, and the
bursar F. Owen Stredder held tight control over the university's business affairs.[32]

At Martin's suggestion, the new principal contributed his voice to
the bid for funding. While paying a visit to another branch of the
Rockefeller Foundation in December, Morgan asked to see Warren
Weaver to establish contact and to talk about the biochemistry department application.[33] Weaver noted in his diary that Morgan impressed
him. The new principal had explained that Collip and Martin had considered that Weaver's letter of 19 September had "closed and locked
the door," but he wanted to inquire "if the door is permanently bolted
or not." Weaver had replied that the foundation had a genuine interest
in Collip's work and recognized the importance of the breadth of his
approach to endocrine problems. He had tactfully suggested, however,
that he and the foundation officers agreed with "the somewhat general
scientific opinion that it will be unfortunate if [Collip] allows his energy, enthusiasm, and imagination to lead him to spread himself too
thin." He had pressed this point further: certain types of expansion to
Collip's program would be a "distinct dis-service to both Collip and to
endocrinology."[34]

Morgan recalled in his own memorandum on the interview that
Weaver had spoken "in terms of highest admiration of Collip and respect for him as a man and a scientist but said that some of his best
friends were nervous lest his great imagination should lead him into
too many fields." The principal recorded that he had come to Collip's
defence, suggesting that while this broad program might in truth be
dangerous for other people, Collip had been able to keep his attention
to his own work; when a project had had multiple ramifications, these
branches were looked after by others. Morgan was left with the sense
that Weaver had accepted this answer, but in Weaver's own record of
the meeting, Morgan's attempt failed to warrant a mention.[35]

At the meeting with Weaver, Morgan also inquired about the foundation's funding policies. Weaver explained that policy had changed
from what it had been in the past. The foundation was no longer interested in funding general science and in building up departments of
fundamental science; instead, it was assisting projects in experimental
biology, particularly those fields that impinged on social problems,

such as the problems of sex, psychiatry, and genetics. Morgan also asked whether an application for a grant would be prejudiced by the fact that an institution had already received several gifts. Weaver admitted that there might be a tendency not to give too much to one place, but that on the other hand, this tendency was outweighed by the fact that the foundation preferred to make grants to an institution with which it was familiar.[36]

Finally, Weaver suggested quite frankly that the succession of requests from McGill had not always been carefully thought through, especially in their financial implications. Weaver also made it clear that the foundation would not be willing to entertain a proposal for expansion that did not clearly and definitely take into account the crucial question of the looming loss of the insulin income after 1940. Morgan conceded that the administrative situation at McGill had been confused and complicated of late, but added quietly and decisively that this period was over. McGill had spoken with several voices and its pronouncements had been confused, but from that point on, it would speak with only one voice. Weaver noted that Morgan gave "every impression of being a most clear-minded and forceful individual."[37]

After their first meeting, Morgan and Weaver continued to correspond about the possibility of Morgan making another visit in the third week of January 1936. There is no record that such a meeting ever happened. If it did not, it may have been because Morgan was experiencing difficulties closer to home. During that year, he had a serious difference of opinion with Beatty and the McGill governors over the question of how the university authorities should deal with the propagation of socialist views by McGill faculty and students. Frost argues that the university was considered to be a centre of socialist scholarship and teaching. Beatty and the governors felt that Morgan was making no effort to ensure that a capitalist view of society was advocated as well. In the Faculty of Medicine, the year 1936 brought the retirement of C.F. Martin, a consequence of the governors of McGill resolving to uphold the regulation that members of staff be retired at the age of sixty-five, a rule that had not been rigorously applied before then. Martin, already several years beyond the limit, was forced to give up his deanship after a remarkable thirteen years in the post. His departure was a great loss to Collip, who had regarded him as a mentor. Martin was succeeded by Grant Fleming.[38]

In September 1936 Collip was invited to be a guest speaker at the grand celebrations for the Harvard Tercentenary. There, he was presented with an honorary doctorate and cited as "a skillful bio-chemist, a bold explorer among the tangled complexities of the internal secretions." At Harvard, he was in the company of distinguished scientists and scholars, including nine Nobel Prize winners; when he presented his paper, he shared the stage with such notable figures as Jean Piaget, Charles Gustav Jung, and Rudolf Carnap. He was asked to participate in a symposium entitled "Factors Determining Human Behaviour" that included talks on the physiological, psychological, and cultural elements that contributed to behaviour. Collip presented a paper about the endocrine factors related to human behaviour and drew upon the work of a number of hormone researchers to suggest the ways in which the actions of the individual might be affected by endocrine activity. He carefully noted that both hereditary factors and the external environment were capable of producing changes in hormone levels.[39]

It is noteworthy that the topic of Collip's paper fell squarely within the bounds of the program that Weaver had devised for the natural science division of the Rockefeller Foundation. This was the only occasion in which Collip so directly dealt with the subject in public. Several years later, Collip responded to some questions that zoologist William Rowan had asked him about possible analogies between races of doves and human races, as characterized by distinct levels of hormone activity. During his years in Alberta, Collip had assisted Rowan in his study of the reproductive biology of migratory birds and had inspired him to investigate the influence of hormones. Collip replied, "This is a subject upon which I have always hesitated to commit myself in print for the reason that I have no firsthand knowledge on it, and also because so much bunk has been written about it." He commented of his Harvard Tercentenary address, "This is as far as I have ever gone in discussing this general subject."[40]

The only further contact that Collip had with the foundation that year was an accidental meeting with F.B. Hanson, Weaver's assistant director, at a lunch table at the Harvard Tercentenary. Hanson recalled in his diary that Collip had inquired about the chances of getting some money for his work, saying that he had a great need for space and that his need would become acute in the future when the insulin royalties ran out. Hanson had been non-committal and had merely suggested that Collip and Morgan should take up the matter with the foundation formally. Hanson noted that Collip had seemed to be under the impression that some definite request was under study by foundation officers or had perhaps been rejected without his knowledge. Upon his return to New York, Hanson inquired about the status of the Collip application and discovered that, as he had expected, no official request was pending. He noted that the position of the foundation was that the "next move was up to Martin." In January of the following year, Weaver officially marked the Collip file dormant: "They to make next approach."[41] Because of misunderstandings and changing priorities, and perhaps because Martin was no longer there to push things forward, that next step was never taken by the McGill group and the long series of negotiations with the Rockefeller Foundation came to naught.

The failure of Collip's proposal was the result of many factors, one of the most significant being that the foundation had simply shifted its priorities from institution building to project grants. The Depression years had begun to have an effect on the income available to the Rockefeller Foundation, and the trustees now insisted that the officers cut back on long-term commitments. This was a situation that foundation officers as well as grant-seekers found extremely frustrating. Alan Gregg, the head of the medical sciences division and a man of broad vision, understood the need to establish and endow several centres of psychiatric and neurological research, but his plans were frequently thwarted by the limitations set by the trustees. He did secure the endowment and grant for the Neurological Institute at McGill in 1932 despite this new emphasis on project grants; the $1,282,652 grant for the institute was the largest appropriation from his division that year, amounting to approximately one-third of his total funds. Between 1935 and 1937 in particular, Gregg felt a growing discontent over the increasing insistence of the trustees that commitments be made for no more than one year. By 1937 he was prepared to tender his resignation over this issue. Wilder Penfield, Gregg's biographer, noted that Gregg was convinced to stay on even though no further institutes were built. In addition to this overall change in foundation policy, the natural sciences division policy also worked against Collip's dream. Robert Kohler argues that although the natural sciences division encouraged cross-disciplinary connections, it did not challenge the traditional departmental and disciplinary boundaries. During these years the foundation was "impervious" to appeals to endow research professorships or to set up special institutes outside the formal departmental structure.[42]

The foundation also rejected Collip's proposal on intellectual grounds. On the surface, Collip's work on the anterior pituitary hormones was a good candidate for funding from the natural sciences division. First, the officers had a great deal of respect for Collip's abilities as a scientist. Although Collip's investigations were not specifically related to human behaviour, Weaver's program was sufficiently broad to include studies of endocrinology, genetics, and other biological sciences that provided an understanding of the physical processes underlying behaviour. Herbert Evans, Collip's competitor in the pituitary field, received funding from the division to the amount of $20,000 per year throughout the 1930s.[43] Weaver's concern was the one expressed by Smith and Engle: Collip was trying to take on too broad a range of problems and was not being sufficiently thorough with any one subject. This was something that Collip was not willing to change. His restless personality expressed itself in this and other aspects of his life. Moreover, throughout his career, he achieved a great deal of success through his habit of "skimming the cream off" one problem and moving quickly on to the next. As the head of a large, enthusiastic group, he was content to allow his associates to follow their own interests rather than tie them to his own projects.

A third factor behind the failure of Collip's application was that it was poorly presented. Martin and Collip neglected to explain the financial implications of their proposal in an open and businesslike manner. Their lack of clarity was partly due to their wish to ask for as much as possible from the foundation and their reluctance to tip their hand too early. In addition, it seems likely that they were hoping, or perhaps gambling, that the foundation would be willing to make up the lost insulin income after 1940. Unfortunately, that was precisely the type of financial commitment that the foundation was no longer willing to make. Further, the new style of grant giving was highly personal. Robert Kohler notes that Weaver was adept at separating his impression of the scientist from his evaluation of the work,[44] but perhaps in this episode, the sometimes unhappy mix of personalities, mishandled meetings, and inaccurate interpretations all contributed to the negative final outcome.

The Rockefeller Foundation continued to support medical research at McGill throughout this period, but only through grants for specific projects. Often these grants were renewed for several years in a row, but commitments were almost always made only one year at a time. Collip's former associates Hans Selye and J.S.L. Browne were the recipients of several foundation grants. Weaver was not averse to considering a broader proposal for the support of endocrinology at McGill, but he remarked in 1937 that "although ... there have been approaches of this sort, they have never come to anything because of a variety of administrative and financial complications."[45]

THE EMMENIN FUND MORTGAGE

Over the next years, Collip's relationship with the administration reflected his deepening dissatisfaction with his institutional position and his desire for greater recognition. As well, his children were growing up and he seems to have felt a need to have his family live in proper style. On 8 April 1937 Collip met with the principal, A.E. Morgan, on his own initiative. Collip was concerned about a number of issues. First, he asked for assurance that if he were to leave McGill, an agreement could be struck so that he could continue to have access to the Emmenin royalties. If this thinly veiled threat were not enough, Collip went on to stress that he had no intention or desire to leave at that time. Morgan agreed that McGill could make the same sort of arrangement for Emmenin that Toronto had for insulin. Next, Collip asked that the royalties be specified as belonging to a department of which he was the head, rather than to the Department of Biochemistry, because he might at some time be assigned to a separate department of endocrinology. Morgan also agreed to this. Collip then talked vaguely about his salary and his $2,500 travel expense account. It seemed to Morgan that Collip was hinting at getting a higher salary, but he did not ask directly, nor did Morgan promise anything. Finally, Collip brought forward a proposal. He argued that this idea had already been under discussion with Sir Arthur Currie and he was certain it would have been carried out if Currie had lived. This was a scheme by which the university would purchase Collip's house and allow him to use it for a nominal rent. Collip even suggested that this might be financially advantageous to the university as it would be able to invest the royalties from Emmenin in real property. Morgan did not discuss the matter seriously at that time but merely indicated that he did not think the Board of Governors would approve such an arrangement. Morgan noted that Collip "did not press it."[46]

Two years earlier, McGill had been given a bequest of four-twentieths of the estate of William G. Cheney, the annual income of which was to be applied to the establishment of a chair or chairs to assist the Faculty of Medicine. Perhaps in part to make up for the disappointing result of the Rockefeller bid, the Board of Governors decided in 1937 to direct the income of $17,000 from the bequest to the biochemistry department for five years and to create the Gilman Cheney Chair of Endocrinology for Collip. Certainly this income helped Collip's financial situation in the short term. A second chair of biochemistry was established for David Thomson.[47]

On 15 April, a week after his meeting with Morgan, Collip wrote two letters to the principal, one to convey his appreciation for the establishment of the Cheney chair[48] and the second to suggest that his department's name be changed from the Department of Biochemistry and Pathology to the Department of Biochemistry and Endocrinology: "In view of the fact that something like ninety per cent of our research work has to do with the general subject of Endocrinology, I have felt in recent years that the department has not been adequately named. The addition of this word 'endocrinology' seems to me to be the most desirable."[49]

Morgan had no opportunity to act on this request. In early April he had become embroiled in an argument with McDonald, Stredder, and Beatty over how much control the principal and the governors should respectively have over the university budget. By 17 April Morgan was forced to resign. Macdonald College vice-principal W.H. Brittain was made acting principal in his place.[50]

During the summer Collip continued to have conversations with the bursar, Owen Stredder, about his proposal that a house be purchased for him. In October Collip pursued the matter with the dean of medicine, Fleming, and the associate dean, Simpson. After some consideration, Fleming and Simpson decided to recommend to the acting principal that the university accede to a modified version of Collip's plan. The Emmenin Fund, under Collip's direction, had accumulated the royalties from the sale of Emmenin for the past several years, and by that date amounted to approximately $28,000. Collip was told that the finance committee was unlikely to entertain a plan to purchase a house for him but might instead allow the university to take up a mortgage on a property that he purchased. The bursar also suggested that the committee might consider a proposal from the dean of medicine that Collip's salary be increased by the amount needed to meet the difference between the carrying charges on the house he presently owned and the one he was to purchase – about $1,500 per annum – provided this increase were to come from the income from the Emmenin Fund. Simpson rationalized: "The productiveness of any man intensively engaged in research is very largely dependent on his freedom from outside worry. The feeling that he is unable to make adequate provision for the well being and comfort of his family is undoubtedly a distraction, which will lessen his value to the institution for which he works." Simpson admitted that there existed no precedent to determine how the Emmenin Fund should be controlled:

The "Emmenin Fund," like certain other special funds which have come to the University through Professor Collip, has, rightly or wrongly, been considered as one which can be expended only on his recommendation. In the absence of any agreement or stipulation to the contrary, precedent would justify him in considering that it may be spent in any way he may desire to further the interests of his department.

He concluded, "It would seem that the Fund could be used quite legitimately for the purpose suggested, and that the net return to the University would be much greater if the money were expended in this way than it would be if it were used for the purchase of equipment and supplies."[51]

By the end of the month, the finance committee had approved the scheme, increasing Collip's salary by $1,500, using the income from the Emmenin Fund first and making up the remainder from the Insulin

Fund. The committee also made it clear that the capital from the Emmenin Fund was to be put under the direct control of the university and that no other expenditures were to be made from it until it had grown sufficiently to provide the full $1,500 as income. The committee approved a loan of $28,000 at an interest rate of 5 per cent from the Emmenin Fund for the special purpose of the purchase of the house for Collip.

With this loan, Collip bought a new house in the prestigious Westmount neighbourhood of Montreal in October 1937. This house, on 622 Sydenham Avenue, was the one after which Collip named his "622" pituitary extract. Collip's daughter recalls that it was very important for her father to get this house: "He wanted a proper place for his family to live." Their home before this had been a modest but adequate semi-detached house. The Sydenham house was grand in comparison, a handsome brick residence with a red tile roof just south of King George Park. It came complete with fifteen rooms, including a conservatory, four bathrooms and a library, where Collip sometimes received his scientific visitors. The house also had seven open fireplaces, a large oak-panelled reception hall, a huge living room, and even a billiard room, where he could indulge in one of his favourite pastimes.[52]

This use of the research fund was unconventional but the dean concluded that it was justified:

I believe it is fair to both parties to assume that payment of $1500 a year is a full recognition of Professor Collip's original contribution in the discovery of the product, and that the royalties beyond the amount necessary to produce this $1500 are paid to the University in return for the publicity value and the use of the University name, and for the relatively small service necessary to maintain the standardization of the product.[53]

BROADER RESPONSIBILITIES

By the end of the decade, larger events intervened to force Collip's focus away from his research enterprise and towards broader issues. In 1938 he was invited to sit on the National Research Council Associate Committee on Medical Research, which was chaired by Fred Banting. The following year, with the start of the war, many scientists at McGill and across the country threw themselves into research projects to support the war effort.[54] Investigations in medical subjects were coordinated and supported by Banting's associate committee. Collip and his laboratory group were among the many who contributed to war research. They investigated such subjects as methods of preserving blood, motion sickness, and traumatic shock. In May of 1940 Frank Blair Hanson of the Rockefeller Foundation ran into Collip by accident while visiting McGill. Collip again expressed concern that his income from the insulin patents had only one year to go. He talked about approaching Alan Gregg for funds the following year unless he should be completely immersed in war research by that time.[55]

It must have been unpleasant for Collip to compare his situation with Penfield's, since the work of the Neurological Institute had continued to garner greater support. In addition to the Rockefeller endowment of $1 million, the institute received many gifts from individual benefactors that were on a much larger scale than the donations that Collip received. From 1935 to 1939, McGill's Board of Governors agreed to subscribe to a guarantee fund in order to balance the university's books. When Sir Herbert S. Holt, one of the governors, was told that he would be given a refund of $16,666.67, Lewis Douglas, Morgan's successor as principal from January 1938, wrote asking Holt whether he might consider returning this amount to the university for its general purposes. Holt agreed to this but specified that he had already promised Penfield $5,000 for his research and noted that he would like to give Collip "something for his research work" as well. While Douglas was somewhat disappointed that these specific gifts would take away from his general funds, he agreed to discuss the matter with Collip and determine what his needs were. When notified of this gift, Collip remarked that the news was a complete surprise to him, since he had never met Sir Herbert and was unaware that he intended to support his work. He immediately telephoned Holt and had a "very pleasant interview" with him. Not one to miss such an opportunity, Collip emphasized that his chief financial concern was not for the immediate present, but for the future of his laboratory. This emphasis turned out to be profitable, as Holt made additional donations to the department in subsequent years. In an interview with the bursar, Collip said that he did not wish to make a claim for any specific amount of the Holt donation, leaving that decision to the principal's discretion. The bursar reported, however, that Collip had "made some intimation that an amount equal to that allocated to Dr. Penfield might be reasonable." The principal suggested to the bursar in a marginal note that "I think perhaps it would be better to make it $3,000."[56]

THE INSULIN PATENTS

The biggest money concern looming in Collip's mind in these years was the end of the insulin royalties, which were set to expire in 1940 or 1941. This money had supported much of Collip's work for the most active decades of his career, and now the income made up more than half his departmental budget. As Lorne Hutchison, the executive secretary of the University of Toronto Insulin Committee commented, when the first agreement had been drawn up in 1923, no one had anticipated that it would operate beyond 1940 or 1941 at the latest. Now, however, new circumstances brought a welcome surprise. University of Toronto researchers had continued to develop insulin in the years since the original discovery, and patents on these processes had also been assigned to the committee. The most notable of these was protamine-zinc insulin, developed by David Scott and A.M. Fisher at the University of Toronto Connaught Medical Research Laboratory between 1935 and 1940. This form of insulin had the advantage of having a longer action than the original insulin. Collip would receive revenue from sales of the original type of insulin as well as for sales of crystalline zinc-insulin and protamine-zinc insulin until 1956, when the last of the patents expired. After that, Lilly provided goodwill grants to Best and Collip, not based on any legal obligations, but out of regard for the friendly relations they had developed over the years. Collip was given a consultantship of $2,500 and his laboratory received a grant of $5,000 annually. This consultantship was to continue until Collip's death and the laboratory grant until three years after that.[57]

F. CYRIL JAMES

In 1939 the principalship of McGill changed hands for the third time in six years. When war threatened in Europe, Lewis Douglas, an American, felt compelled to resign and return to the United States. There, he became the first director of the War Shipping Administration and later the U.S. ambassador to Britain. He was succeeded by F. Cyril James, an Englishman who was professor of finance and economic history at the University of Pennsylvania. Douglas had initially appointed James to reorganize the McGill School of Commerce, but James arrived in Montreal on 3 September, the day Britain declared war. Seven days later, Canada declared war on her own. By the end of the following month, the McGill board asked James to assume the principalship. James was to hold this position for the next twenty years. McGill's historian Stanley Frost remarks that James ran "a very efficient, tightly geared, almost one-man operation." James quickly attained dominance in university affairs, a development helped by the absence of the chancellor, Beatty, after a serious illness in 1939. While James acknowledged the authority of the board, he gradually made it clear that authority was to be exercised through his office.[58]

BANTING'S MANTLE

In the two decades since the insulin discovery and the attending turmoil among the discoverers, Banting and Best had become increasingly estranged. Initially, comfortable in his role of hero and senior to his student assistant, Banting had amply rewarded Best's loyalty by championing his claim to credit for the insulin work. Over the years, however, Best had grown from a stalwart young assistant to a fine researcher in his own right, and had therefore become a challenge to Banting. Banting and Best, both at the University of Toronto, began to chafe at the bond that would forever link their names and seat them next to each other at commemorative events. Banting, whose research skills were limited, struggled vainly to find another great cure and to live up to the hopes invested in him by so many institutions and individuals who supported his research. Best, over the years, may have become less and less willing to take second place to someone whom he had increasingly come to view as his inferior as a research scientist.[59]

On the other hand, Banting and Collip had become close friends after their early legendary fights. One story has the two of them meeting again at the Calgary Stampede sometime in the mid-1930s, an event that was recorded by Collip's young son Jack, a keen photographer. Banting brought Collip to work with him on the National Research Council medical research committee, and Collip served as his assistant chairman from 1938. In February 1941 Banting stopped on his way through Montreal to see Collip before heading overseas on a war-related mission. Michael Bliss describes the warm conversation they had in Banting's hotel room, reliving their insulin days. Collip noticed Banting was without warm gloves when he took him to the airport and insisted that he take his own sheepskin gloves. As Banting's plane flew over Newfoundland, it crashed, killing Banting and two others.[60]

Collip was badly shaken by the news of Banting's death. His colleague George Hunter at the Department of Biochemistry at the University of Alberta wrote him of the accident: "Its [sic] the worst disaster in Canadian history ... His mantle is going to fall on both Charlie Best and you: the mantle of responsibility in maintaining medical research in Canada."[61]

Later that year, Collip won the Charles Mickle Fellowship of the University of Toronto. Banting's faithful assistant Sadie Gairns wrote Collip with her congratulations, saying she felt that Banting would have been very pleased. She added that she was appalled that Best had been named as the "obvious successor" to Banting's chair at the Banting and Best Department of Medical Research at Toronto. She told

Collip that she had even gone so far as to tell the president that "it was the last person Dr. Banting would want to succeed him."[62]

THE RESEARCH INSTITUTE OF ENDOCRINOLOGY

Collip renewed his efforts to have a research institute established in 1941. Perhaps he was responding to the fact that Best now had charge of his own research department. Perhaps he felt that he bore Banting's mantle and thus deserved greater institutional recognition. Or, perhaps Banting's death had signalled to him his own mortality. The arrival of the new principal brought a new opportunity to bring forward the proposal.

Many years later, after Collip's death, James candidly recalled his acute observations and very definite view of Collip in 1941:

Bert was an extraordinarily poor departmental chairman, interested primarily in his own researches and in those of the graduate students who happened to impinge on his own special interests ... This fact led me to feel that somehow or other we should find a way of switching Bert Collip from the important departmental chairmanship into a job appropriate to his prestige and talents but removed from the whole question of under-graduate teaching – both in Medicine and in Arts and Sciences.[63]

James was presented with a solution to this problem when Collip expressed his wish for a research institute of endocrinology, one comparable to the Neurological Institute. James promptly seized on the idea and set about making it work out administratively, even though the university finances were very straitened at the time.[64]

In August 1941 the Board of Governors set up the Research Institute of Endocrinology. The terms were most generous. It was first understood that Collip would take the income from the insulin, Emmenin, and Pituitrin royalties with him to the new institute. Furthermore, the university provided $7,000 towards physical reconstruction and moving expenses. Collip was appointed director of the institute but retained his Gilman Cheney professorship, which came with a substantial annual income of $17,000. In an attempt to reach a somewhat more equitable and gradual readjustment of the financial arrangements between the new institute and the Department of Biochemistry (and probably to avoid impoverishing the department entirely), it was determined that the whole of the Cheney income would not be given to the institute. Instead, provision was made so that whenever Collip's insulin income exceeded $10,000, then $8,500 of the Cheney funds would be transferred back to Biochemistry. If, however, the insulin income fell below $10,000, the Cheney funds would be used to make up the difference and the department would get what was left. This gave Collip a guarantee of a sizable annual income: $17,000 from the Cheney bequest, at least $10,000 from insulin, and $4,000 from Emmenin and Pituitrin, minus the $8,500 to Biochemistry. However, the university was not prepared to provide the institute with more than the Cheney income. James hoped that since Collip and his staff were becoming increasingly preoccupied with war research and because so many of his projects were now funded by the government, perhaps he and his staff would not need to use that full amount. In a letter to Collip, James wrote that he shared Collip's wish that, instead, enough income could be set aside to build up an endowment that would ensure the stability of research funding in the future.[65]

Collip's new institute occupied the west wing of the Medical Building, the former location of the Public Health Department. While the rooms were old, they were light and airy and, most importantly, large enough to accommodate four or five researchers plus technicians.[66] In leaving the biochemistry department, Collip took with him Robert Noble and Abe Neufeld as his senior assistants. David Thomsom stayed on in Biochemisty and took over as the head of the department. Collip gave his graduate students and staff the option of joining his institute or remaining in the department. All chose to go with him except Orville Denstedt, who remained with Thomson.

In addition to taking most of the staff and funds with him, Collip also took much of the equipment. Even as late as 1950, members of the biochemistry department were still trying to make up for the loss. At that time, Denstedt negotiated with the university to buy a large used refrigerator that had been standing dismantled for three or four years and that the university had been thinking of selling to the Faculty Club. In a rather pitiful letter, Denstedt had to explain that the department had been without a large refrigerator in the several years since Collip had left and that, as a result, the researchers had been forced to curtail their work on proteins for lack of adequate refrigeration.[67]

After 1941 Collip succeeded Banting as the chairman of the NRC Associate Committee on Medical Research. During the final years of the war, he found himself ever more preoccupied with administrative responsibilities. His outlook changed, too, broadening out from his own research problems to the concerns of organizing medical research across the country. Ironically, now that he was finally established in his hard-won new post as research professor, he spent more time away from his laboratory than ever. He was grateful, though, that since his chair came with no specific teaching responsibilities, he was able to devote his time and energies to wartime committee work without causing a serious disruption.[68]

However, all these new responsibilities and honours seemed not to be enough for Collip. Only a year after he won his institute, he had a frank discussion with James, expressing his interest in the position of dean of graduate studies. After some consideration, James wrote to Collip, telling him that he was going to appoint David Thomson to the office instead. James explained his rationale: "I feel more strongly than ever that it would be contrary to the best interest of the University if we should regard appointment to any deanship as a reward for scholarly merit." A deanship to him was clearly an administrative office and required someone who could be available at all times to pay attention to routine details and to undertake "a lot of donkey work." It required someone who was willing to put the university at the centre of his career. James noted pointedly that it was necessary for the dean to be familiar with teaching. He gently suggested that

when the war is over, and you are able to lay down the heavy burden of National Research Council work which you have so generously undertaken in the public interest, your scientific eminence and your detailed knowledge of the Canadian scene in matters of scientific research would make you an outstanding candidate for the Deanship, the present moment, however, I feel that those wider activities would be a handicap to you in dealing with the domestic problems of the University ... I hope that you will, on reflection, realize that this decision is in no sense a reflection upon your own scientific eminence, of which I and all your colleagues are very proud.[69]

The war meant the total disruption of the work of the new endocrinology institute. Collip's own energies were devoted to the administrative work of the NRC and to serving as Canada's medical liaison officer for the United States. He spent much of the period travelling between Ottawa and Washington, making stops in Montreal whenever possible. Abe Neufeld had taken a position as a resident liaison officer in the Office of the U.S. Surgeon General in Washington.

In Montreal, Bob Noble plunged himself into war research. One dramatic addition to the institute was a large swing he built to study motion sickness, a problem faced by sailors and airmen, paratroops and commandos. Noble contributed a considerable amount of research on the use of barbiturates to treat the problem.[70] In biochemistry, Orville Denstedt produced important work on the storage of human blood and devised a method of preserving whole blood for six to eight weeks. Blood donated by volunteers was preserved according to his procedure and shipped overseas to Britain after the invasion of Europe, though never in quantities sufficient for clinical use.[71] Collip and Noble also conducted some research on the use of cortical extracts to prevent or alleviate shock. Noble's inventive mind even led him into fields that were not much related to medical science. Fascinated by the problem of the movement of troops across stretches of muddy countryside, Noble developed mud-shoes, something of a cross between snowshoes and skis. He filmed trials of his prototype in action on the muddy clay of McGill's grounds, as well as in Greenwich, Connecticut.[72]

After the war, a Rockefeller officer once again visited Collip at McGill. During his visit, R.S. Morison, an assistant director under Alan Gregg, gained the distinct impression that the Research Institute of Endocrinology had never really gotten going. Collip was still very much involved with the NRC war committees, and it seemed likely he would be made director of any peacetime committee of the council that might be established. Morison noted that Collip seemed to harbour feelings of annoyance for Warren Weaver, believing that Weaver had somehow blocked a Rockefeller grant for his proposed addition to the Biological Building some ten years earlier. Since Morison had not known the details of the case, he had simply tried to explain to Collip that "bricks and mortar" expenditures had stopped just about that time as a matter of policy. Concerned, Morison related this conversation to Weaver when he returned to the Rockefeller. In answer to his questions, Weaver gave him the decade-old file on Collip's application. After studying the file, Morison wrote to Weaver, "I had suspected that [Collip's] intensity of feeling was greater than his knowledge on this point," and concluded, "and the prophesy of his spreading himself too thin seems to have been pretty amply fulfilled."[73]

Once the war was over, Collip found it difficult to settle into research work again. Finding the research facilities in his new institute inadequate, he began to discuss proposals for expansion with the brothers Samuel and Allan Bronfman of the Seagrams distillery fortune. Sam Bronfman had given generously to McGill for many years in his attempt to gain an invitation to sit on the Board of Governors, an entree into in Montreal's Anglo society. According Michael Marrus, Bronfman's biographer, Bronfman found himself excluded from the board because of strong anti-Semitic sentiments at McGill and particularly because of the personal opposition of J.W. McConnell, then the publisher of the *Montreal Star* and McGill's most generous benefactor. Bronfman had to wait until 1965, after McConnell's death, to reach his goal.[74]

During this period, Collip worked with the Bronfmans to develop a plan for the construction of additional laboratory facilities at McGill's Macdonald College at Ste-Anne-de-Bellevue on the western end of the Island of Montreal. Macdonald College was the home of McGill's agricultural school and the School of Household Science. The proposed new building was intended to enable Collip and his staff to carry out

larger-scale experiments than were possible in the Medical Building. By
1947 plans for the Macdonald campus building were so advanced that
Bob Noble and his family bought a house out at Ste-Anne-de Bellevue
in preparation for the move.[75]

A FRESH START:
THE UNIVERSITY OF WESTERN ONTARIO

At the same time, a very different proposal was presented to Collip.
G.E. Hall was about to leave his position as dean of medicine at the
University of Western Ontario (UWO) to take up the presidency at the
university. Ed Hall was a medical scientist and a former protegé of
Banting's. He was also a friend and long-time admirer of Collip's and
the two had worked together on the wartime committees of the NRC.
During the war, Hall had written to him: "Your contributions to the
Council itself have been great and many of us recognize just how much
you have put into making the whole Medical Research aspects of the
NRC an international success. Our appreciation for your work is un-
bounded and I express the feelings of many."[76]

Now, the ambitious Hall hoped to turn this friendly connection into
a real coup for Western; he offered Collip the deanship of medicine as
well as an appointment as head of a new department of medical research. Hall had great plans for his university, and bringing a scientist
of Collip's stature to head the medical school was a bold move.

With his research institute in place and his plans for expansion with
the Bronfmans already underway, not many would have expected Collip to be tempted by this invitation. Not only would he be moving from
a research position to an administrative one, he would be going from
one of the two top universities in the country to a much less prestigious
school. The Collip of 1947, though, may have been quite a different
man from the one he had been in the prewar days when he had been
rivetted to his bench, the happy centre of activity in his lab. With the
war over, Collip found it difficult to return to research with the same
vigour he had had before. The Rockefeller's Morison had even ventured this opinion in his notes: "I should take even money that his own
research days are over." In 1948 Collip admitted in a draft of a lecture,
"I find it extremely difficult, after a lapse of so many years in which I
have been engaged in administrative duties for the most part, to discuss
research problems, the pursuit of which, in a personal way, I have now
been so far removed."[77]

Collip may also have been dissatisfied with the recognition he had
received at McGill. J.C. Meakins was retiring that year, vacating his
post as dean of medicine, and some suggested that Collip aspired to

succeed him. Certainly Collip had expressed his interest in becoming dean of graduate studies several years earlier. Finally, after spending several years involved in questions of organizing medical research, Collip began to feel that he had some experience to offer in this area. He thought he might want to take on the new challenge of administering a medical school. Collip explained in a letter to Charles Martin and his wife that having been at McGill for nineteen years, he was wary of the problems associated with a large, prominent medical school. He noted pointedly that he was especially concerned with the uncoordinated growth of the various departments and the favouritism shown to certain divisions. Thus, the University of Western Ontario offer presented an opportunity to start afresh and try out his own ideas about running a medical faculty.[78]

By March, Collip began to give hints that he was considering the move. He wrote to James requesting a formal statement about the disposition of his various research funds should he move to another medical school. He suggested that if such a move were to happen, the Insulin Fund should be transferred with him *in toto*. Royalties for the products he had developed at McGill might be split, one half to remain at McGill and the other half to go with him to his new institution. One month later, Hall was able to present Collip with an official offer. At this stage, Collip spoke with James and told him frankly of the offer from Western. The McGill board agreed with Collip's reasoning that the entire Insulin Fund, which he had brought to McGill with him, should be transferred with him, but that half the accumulated capital and half the future revenues of the Emmenin, Pituitrin, and Premarin funds should remain at McGill. In a letter to Collip in April, James agreed that he could see the attraction of the uwo offer, but protested, "I am still of the opinion that with the developments which we have discussed and foreshadowed, you would find yourself even happier at McGill University during the next decade."[79]

Collip's associates Bob Noble and Don Heard were offered appointments at Western as well, as professor and associate professor respectively. Noble, despite the fact that he and his wife had already purchased a home near Macdonald College, decided to follow Collip. Heard, a talented steroid chemist, chose to turn down the offer from Western as well as another tempting offer from an American research institute in order to stay at McGill. Hall wrote to notify James that these offers had been made, and James replied:

It is scarcely necessary for me to say that you would be very fortunate indeed if you were able to persuade [Collip] to accept such an appointment but, to reciprocate your frankness, I had told Dr. Collip that I should like to see him remain at McGill University and shall do all that I can to encourage him to reach that decision. He is so popular a member of the Medical Faculty and so distinguished a scientist that his departure would leave a very uncomfortable vacancy in our ranks.[80]

Collip's mind had already been made up. He had decided to go to London.

The news that Collip had accepted the appointment at Western came as a shock to many of his friends and associates at McGill. Many called the loss of such an outstanding scientist a terrible blow to McGill's reputation. James had been very occupied with the task of building a strong academic staff and had been able to make numerous junior appointments to various departments, but none of the new staff had yet proved themselves and certainly none had yet attained the stature of someone like Collip. W.W. Chipman, a governor and a past associate of Collip's, telephoned the principal to ask for an explanation of Collip's departure. He demanded that James explain how he had failed to prevent this great loss to McGill. James defended himself, arguing that he had helped to create the Research Institute of Endocrinology for Collip, giving the scientist an organization over which he had full control. Collip had also always had ample funds. In the years since his arrival, Collip's royalty income had brought close to three-quarters of a million dollars to McGill, more than half from insulin and the remainder from Emmenin, Premarin, and Pituitrin. James argued, "That there was not shortage of money is indicated by the fact that the University will have to transfer very substantial funds to the University of Western Ontario when Collip leaves us." Indeed, Collip took some $160,000 with him to Western. James further explained that he had been working over the past year with Collip and the Bronfmans on plans for the research laboratories at Macdonald College. The Bronfmans had agreed only a few weeks before to pay approximately $100,000 for the construction. James had even assured Collip that if he could be encouraged to stay on, he could have anything he wanted "within reasonable limits."[81]

James offered the opinion that Collip had decided to go to London because he and his wife wanted to live in a smaller centre. As well, Collip had developed many ideas on the philosophy of medical education, and he wanted to try his hand at being dean of a medical school with a small student body and faculty. When James had been considering a successor to Meakins as dean of medicine, he had consulted with Collip. According to James, Collip had stated definitely that he would not under any circumstances accept the post, since the McGill medical faculty was too large and amorphous and had all the problems of keeping several large departments together along with the difficulties of maintaining relations with two teaching hospitals. James concluded his explanation by detailing the generous financial provisions that McGill had made for Collip, from his handsome salary, to the items purchased for his private library out of research funds, to the large mortgage on his house in Westmount, for which he had not been asked for capital repayments.[82]

Collip's own rationale for the move is suggested in a letter he wrote to Charles Martin, the man who had brought him to McGill many years before: "I thought I would be a fixture there for the rest of my active days and if fate had been sufficiently kind to have allowed you to remain my mentor, I feel quite sure that such would have been the case, all in all however I must admit that McGill hasn't treated me too badly but things could never be or have they been the same after you relinquished the Deanship of Medicine." He commented on the surprise generated by his announcement:

I rather fear that some of my friends, not conversant with all the circumstances will feel that I am taking a backward step but of this I personally have no misgivings as I am completely satisfied that in the theoretical ten years of service that remain to me I should be able to contribute vastly more to the field of Med. R. and teaching than I possibly could at McGill quite irrespective of the rosy picture which the Principal has endeavored to paint for me with the added privilege so to speak of writing my own ticket.

He continued:

The one thing that gives me most concern is the possibility that this move may be considered as something of "sour grapes." The deanship of Medicine at McGill today holds no attraction whatever for me as you will doubtless be well able to understand. I think Fred Smith in agreeing to accept this post is doing it entirely out of a sense of duty and self sacrifice for all of which he has my profound admiration and should I have decided to remain at McGill there is probably no other person who could have been selected for this post with whom I could be in so much sympathy.

Collip also talked candidly about the disappointments he had experienced with research at his institute:

As I recall it you never showed any great enthusiasm on my transfer from the chair of my first home at McGill in which you and Sir Arthur installed me in 1928 to the so called Institute of Endocrinology. Looking back at it now, I realize all too well how right you were as I now consider the latter to have been an abortion from the start. There probably was no other way to solve the exigencies that arose as a result of the war and I should be eternally grateful for the fact that this move allowed me to give practically full time to government service. No Endocrine work of any significance has been done in this Institute but I must say I am very proud of the contributions which the staff were able to make in so called war research. In going therefore to be chair of M.R. you will, I am sure understand that I cannot have many regrets at leaving the top floor of the west wing of the Medical building now so hopelessly inadequate for modern laboratory space. The alternative to this you know was to build another institute at St. Anne's (with the help of Mr. Bronfman). Strange to say or perhaps not so strange I have never been able to get very enthusiastic about this latter project.

Thus this new post would offer a fresh start:

At London on the other hand the situation is almost ideal. It's a small school strictly limited to 60 students per year. The departments for the most part staffed by young men in their thirties with already proven abilities, with fine personalities and a cooperative spirit which would do your heart good to see. The Med library is one of the best in Canada, a brand new 600 bed hospital is just across the street from the teaching and research labs and there is the closest cooperation between the surgical and medical dept. and all of these. It really gives me a great thrill to see all of this and to realize that it will be up to me to integrate and greatly expand the whole program there. It is my intention to so develop in as far as I am able the dept of M.R. (which by the way has been stripped bare for my inheritance so that there is no dead wood to be dealt with) so that it will fit into the picture as a whole supporting and collaborating with all of the pre-clinical as well as the clinical departments so that the school should go forward as a whole rather than in the favoured development in special parts. I know that it may be hard to keep to this ideal but I have seen enough of the opposite at McGill in the mushroom spawning of specialized labs uncoordinated and unrelated to any external policy.[83]

Comments from colleagues were mixed. Harold Ettinger of Queen's University framed the appointment as a coup for Hall and Western: "This is the most important challenge that Ed has yet thrown at the other Ontario Medical Schools." C.J. Mackenzie, president of the NRC, remarked, "I have no doubt that from your personal standpoint you will find the change not only pleasant but exhilarating, and we are all looking forward to great things to come out of Western." Other friends were less enthusiastic and commented that they did not know whether to offer congratulations or not. A Montreal associate reported that the news of Collip's departure was the general topic of conversation at lunch at the University Club and that no one was happy to know that he was leaving. Collip was grateful to have one friend who fully appreciated the opportunities he felt this offered him. Charles Mitchell, animal pathologist at the Department of Agriculture, had served with Collip on NRC committees and wrote:

It seems to me that you will be placed in a position which will give scope for the organization of medical training and medical research and that when you quit the post some years hence a legacy will be left behind of better facilities for undergraduate and postgraduate training. It is regrettable that McGill should lose your services. I know that much of the fame of the medical school of McGill University at the present time is the result of your research. Too often Universities overlook the capacity of workers for organizing research on a wider field and which actually gives more scope for activities on a wider plane.[84]

When Collip moved to London, in addition to taking much of the research funding with him, he also took a great deal of the equipment that had been purchased over the years out of the various research funds. The residue of the funds at McGill were made into a Collip Research Fund that provided grants and scholarships for research in the pre-clinical sciences. Ayerst, McKenna and Harrison, having developed a long association with Collip, devised a scheme to divert more of their support to Western. Likely in consultation with Collip, Ayerst renegotiated its agreement with McGill. Instead of royalties, Ayerst offered to pay a fixed annual sum. This sum was less than half the amount the university gained through its royalties, and as the McGill bursar suspected, Ayerst then took the amount saved and donated it to the University of Western Ontario for Collip's work. But as David Thomson noted ruefully, McGill was in no position to argue. It no longer contributed to controlling the manufacture of Emmenin, nor was the use of the McGill name likely to be of as much value to the firm as it had been in the early years. More importantly, Collip took his strong research reputation with him to Western.

At McGill, J.S.L. Browne continued to produce important work in clinical endocrinology at the Royal Victoria Hospital. David Thomson was appointed to the Gilman Cheney chair and remained head of the biochemistry department and dean of graduate studies. Thomson, who had always been at his best as a teacher and later as an administrator, was too occupied with his other duties to personally continue the research tradition. Thomson urged the principal to try to hang on to Don Heard, who had been receiving invitations from other institutions. Thomson argued that Heard, a steroid chemist with an international reputation, "can do much to prevent McGill from losing the fame it has long had as a source of leadership in Endocrinology."[85]

SUSTAINING A RESEARCH ENTERPRISE

During his years at McGill, Collip had developed a research enterprise that had few equals in Canada. He successfully built his career on the dual legacy of his insulin achievement – an international reputation and a substantial royalty income. One of the chief needs of his Canadian research contemporaries was a reliable source of funding. Collip was able to secure this through his royalties, first from insulin and later from Emmenin, Premarin, and, with less success, Pituitrin. A sizable portion of his research program was devoted to developing therapeutically valuable products. While Collip may have been motivated by the wish to make a contribution as dramatic as insulin, he was certainly also well aware that the commercial success of such products could help to support a research program. He very actively promoted the commercial development of his many hormone extracts.

Like other researcher-entrepreneurs of this era, he also solicited the aid of private individuals and philanthropic foundations. As one of the more renowned scientists in Canada, Collip was able to attract the interest of a number of patrons. While he resented having to take time from his researches, he knew the importance of cultivating personal relationships with wealthy benefactors. Seeking foundation support was a complicated matter that involved strategies and perseverance. That Collip was seriously considered for a major Rockefeller Foundation grant speaks to his eminence as a scientist, his abilities as laboratory chief, and the importance and currency of his work on pituitary hormones. That his bid failed reflects the incompatibility of his aims with those of the foundation, their differing views on the scope of his research program, as well as more mundane problems of administration. While Collip was willing to play up the behavioural implications of his studies to some extent, he was unwilling, or perhaps unable, to change his broadly focused approach to the field.

As one of McGill's most distinguished scientists, Collip was in a good position to negotiate with the university. In the most active phase of his research career, his concerns centred on gaining a stable source of funding and a release from teaching and administrative duties. When the Rockefeller application failed, the medical faculty was able to divert money from a large general endowment to his department. His unusually comfortable position of having authority over sizable research funds put the university in the very unorthodox position of having to authorize a mortgage for his private home out of money designated for research purposes and then having to justify the arrangement as a means of securing a happier employee.

Later, as government work took Collip away from the research bench, he aspired to gain greater recognition in other ways. He seems to have regarded the deanship of graduate studies, at least in part, as an appropriate reward for his research achievements. While documents of 1947 (James's letter to Chipman and Collip's own vigorous protest to Martin) seem to indicate that Collip did not desire the deanship of medicine at McGill, later material at least suggests that he had been ambivalent. James recalled in 1965, just after Collip's death, that he had felt that Collip was quite happy with his position at the Research Institute, but that "as he approached the age of retirement (rather like Penfield) he did not wish to retire and was rather annoyed at the suggestion that he was not different from all the other members of the staff." James also remembered: "It was only in our discussions after his appointment [at Western] that I realised he had long cherished the idea that he would make an ideal Dean of the Faculty of Medicine at McGill. I may be wrong, but I think that it would have been a calamitous appointment for us, although I think he did reasonably well at Western with a smaller Faculty and a medical scientist as President of the University."[86] The lengths to which the medical faculty and the university went to accommodate Collip indicate how valuable his work and reputation were to them in maintaining the strong medical tradition.

At the close of the war, perhaps recognizing that his best research days were behind him, Collip decided that it would be best to use his years of knowledge and experience in a different way. It became apparent that he desired something that McGill could no longer provide – a place in which he could start anew and try out the ideas he had been cultivating over many years. In choosing the deanship at the University of Western Ontario, he was perhaps accepting a role befitting not a scientist in his prime, but an elder statesman of medical research in Canada.

7

The Rise of Public Funding, 1938–1968:
Medical Research on a National Level

Medical research in Canada is at the critical stage ... I believe that this discussion that we have had today is extremely important inasmuch as it is passing on to the government the responsibility for medical research. Today will go down in our history as marking an epoch; we have taken a step in the right direction.

Sir Frederick Banting, Conference on the Organization of Medical Research in Canada, 18 February 1938[1]

Since his days as a graduate student at the University of Toronto, Collip had been a dedicated scientist who loved nothing more than working away at some new problem late into the night. He had continually struggled to arrange his working conditions so that he could devote himself exclusively to research. His perspective on medical research began to broaden, however, when he accepted the invitation to sit on the National Research Council's Associate Committee on Medical Research in 1938. Collip's colleagues were surprised by how enthusiastically he took to the intensive committee work because he had previously shown very little interest in administrative matters.[2] His involvement with the medical research arm of the NRC stretched over the next twenty years and became one of his primary occupations. In shaping policy, he drew from his own experiences in the world of science. While his glory days at the bench were now over, he was able to support those who followed by helping to establish the systematic funding of medical research activities in Canada.

For most of Collip's career, he had funded the research of his laboratory through private means. The most significant source of funds was the royalties from therapeutic products that he had helped to develop, such as insulin, Emmenin, and Premarin. Collip also received some grants from philanthropic foundations and private benefactors. Towards the end of his career, he saw the burden of financing medical research pass to the government and, indeed, helped to shepherd in this new development. His well-established research enterprise at McGill was a prime candidate for public funds. He and his laboratory group were among the first to benefit from government grants.

The funding and coordination of medical research officially became a governmental responsibility in Canada when the National Research Council established its Associate Committee on Medical Research in 1938. Medical research was fostered by the NRC from that point on until 1960, when the independent Medical Research Council was created. The policies and practices developed by the Associate Committee and its successor, the Division of Medical Research, helped to institutionalize and shape the growth of Canadian medical science.[3]

The early members of the Associate Committee struggled with the problem of how to promote research on a national basis. Institutional support for research was generally low in Canadian universities of this period. Academic scientists often carried heavy teaching loads and lacked sufficient funds to hire assistants or purchase equipment. Furthermore, investigators, particularly those outside Toronto and Montreal, experienced intellectual isolation from their scientific peers. Finally, aspiring Canadian students found insufficient opportunities and support for post-graduate study and too few academic posts once they had completed their education. The result was that many promising young graduates were lost through emigration to the United States, where prospects for careers in medical science were greater.[4]

The policies and practices established during the early years of the Associate Committee and the Division of Medical Research shaped the growth of medical research. Unlike its counterparts in the United States and Britain, which created central laboratories, the Canadian committee chose to develop a system of support that was entirely extramural. As a result, medical research was characterized by a particularly close connection with medical schools. The committee also actively promoted the development of centres of research outside of the older, more established institutions in central Canada. Its hope was to have medical research develop on a more even basis across the country.[5]

In 1916 the National Research Council of Canada was created to advise the government and to promote industrial research. One of its first actions was to set up a system of studentships and fellowships to support post-graduate studies in the sciences and a set of grants-in-aid for established investigators. Yves Gingras credits the post-graduate support program with the institutionalization of the scientific research capacity of universities. These awards were made primarily to students in physics and chemistry. During its first twenty-two years, the NRC did not accept responsibility for medical research in any general way, though it supported important work on specific projects, most notably the study of tuberculosis. This was the case despite the fact that the first chairman of the NRC was Collip's mentor, biochemist A.B. Macallum.[6]

Canadian medical scientists in the early decades of the century had little in the way of financial support from their home institutions. By 1920 both McGill and the University of Toronto, the only two universities with fully developed graduate programs, had begun to set aside university funds to support research. Other sources were available as well; for example, proceeds from the sale of sera and antitoxins by the University of Toronto's Connaught Antitoxin Laboratories were put towards research. By 1920 the Connaught research fund had amassed over $100,000.[7]

It was the exception to be able to generate funds for medical research from patent royalties. The royalties that Banting, Best, and Collip shared with the general research fund of the University of Toronto garnered an average of over $180,000 a year during the 1930s, constituting one of the largest pools of money in support of medical science in Canada. The insulin proceeds had been a very secure and unusually bountiful base from which Collip had been able to launch the rest of his research career. Another legacy of the insulin discovery was the Banting Research Foundation, which provided grants and fellowships to medical investigators. As well, American philanthropic foundations such as the Rockefeller Foundation and the Carnegie Corporation funnelled millions of dollars into medical education and research in this country.[8]

In 1936, when Banting was asked to serve on the National Research Council, he agreed to do so on the condition that medical research be funded on the same basis as the other sciences. In November of that year, Banting worked with NRC president A.G.L. McNaughton to draft a proposal for the organization of medical research. Their chief recommendation was the establishment of an associate committee on medical research, and their vision of its functions indicates that they favoured vigorous government involvement in research. They argued that while a considerable amount of work was being conducted, some of it of great merit, "full value" was not being obtained because no central body was available to coordinate the activities. They felt that such a body could survey the field, ensure that investigations were assigned to those who were best qualified and equipped to carry them out, and correlate the results obtained. Banting and McNaughton suggested that $7,500 be made available for the preliminary organization of the committee. During the early stages of planning, they assumed that the main function of the committee would be one of correlating rather than funding research. General McNaughton expressed the opinion that while no provision had yet been made for the financial support of the committee, "his experience had been that funds were always forthcoming when the needs were properly established and adequately presented."[9]

Banting and McNaughton then solicited the opinions of the Canadian Medical Association (CMA), the Royal College of Physicians and Surgeons, and the federal government's Department of Pensions and National Health. The response was largely positive, with many looking towards the British Medical Research Council as a model. The members of the CMA executive demonstrated "an overwhelming opinion in favour of" the idea of the committee and "a fervent hope ... that this would the first step toward the establishment of a Medical Research Council for Canada similar in scope and function to the Medical Research Council of the United Kingdom." R.E. Wodehouse, deputy minister of the Department of Pensions and National Health, was even more vigorous in his support. In private conversation, McNaughton noted that Wodehouse advocated organizing a separate council immediately rather than proceeding through intermediate stages. Furthermore, in place of the rather modest budget suggested by Banting and McNaughton, he was in favour of asking for at least $50,000 to $100,000 for the first year. McNaughton and CMA representatives, however, opted for more a more cautious strategy, as they felt that the new organization had to gain the confidence of the medical profession and that this was best achieved through a more gradual approach.[10]

Although positive responses predominated, researchers were not uniformly enthusiastic. J.G. FitzGerald, director of both the University of Toronto School of Hygiene and Connaught Laboratories, shared his reservations about the proposal. He was concerned that there were already too many associations for organizing research and that the small number of investigators in the country were already spending too much of their time at meetings and looking after administrative details and not enough engaged in research.[11]

In February of the following year, McNaughton followed up on this consultation by convening a general conference of representatives of every institution and organization across the country with an interest in medical research – universities with departments or faculties of medicine, universities with pre-medical courses, research institutions outside universities, provincial departments of health, and national organizations concerned with medicine. The task of the conference was to nominate the personnel and outline the scope and duties of the committee. T.H. Leggett, president of the CMA, expressed his objectives of securing greater funds for research and encouraging younger workers.[12]

By this date, Wodehouse had come to agree that the interests of the medical profession would be served best by not making an attempt to set up an independent council immediately. Nevertheless, at the conference, he continued to express concern about having the medical research body tied to the NRC. Saying he was speaking not in his official capacity but "as a medical man with medical man's interests," he suggested that these interests "could possibly be jeopardized unknowingly by people whose intentions were of the best." While he expressed friendly feelings towards the NRC, he believed that it would be preferable for the proposed organization to be autonomous, just as its counterparts were in England, the United States, South Africa, Australia, and France. McNaughton hastened to assure him that the NRC considered the creation of the committee to be only a preliminary measure and that when an autonomous council became necessary, the NRC would give it every assistance.[13]

Representatives from across Canada reported on the work being conducted at their institutions. The primary theme that emerged from their presentations was the pressing need for funds. At the close of the session, Banting described his vision of medical research. Research could no longer be regarded as a luxury that might be run on the charity of private benefactors, but as an enterprise of national importance, deserving of governmental support:

I think we are all surprised at the scope and amount of medical research that is actually being carried on in Canada. Medical research in Canada is at the critical stage. For the most part it has been carried on by wealthy people. In this day of high taxation it is becoming increasingly difficult to obtain funds from individuals. I believe that this discussion that we have had today is extremely important inasmuch as it is passing on to the government the responsibility for medical research. Today will go down in our history as marking an epoch; we have taken a step in the right direction.[14]

Delegates debated a number of questions, such as how to determine the relative support that should go to laboratory and clinical research, whether support should be directed towards established centres or less-developed ones, and whether to create central laboratories or to promote research at existing institutions. The report of the conference concluded with the recommendation that the NRC create an associate committee with terms of reference very much like those Banting and McNaughton had drawn up:

a) To receive suggestions for requirements in respect of medical research and in matters related thereto.
b) To consider by whom the investigations required can best be carried out and to make proposals accordingly.
c) To correlate the information when secured and to make it available to those concerned.
d) To do such other things as the Committee may deem advisable to promote medical research in Canada.[15]

THE ASSOCIATE COMMITTEE
ON MEDICAL RESEARCH

In 1938 the Associate Committee on Medical Research was created with Banting as its chair. Collip was appointed to the committee soon after. The first act of the Associate Committee was to conduct a survey of the existing facilities for medical research. Banting, accompanied by Chester Stewart, the assistant secretary of the committee, travelled across the country making personal visits to every medical school and major hospital, to the pre-medical departments of those universities with no medical school, and to provincial laboratories of the departments of public health. They met and interviewed some three hundred workers, including those in Collip's laboratory at McGill. Banting concluded, not surprisingly, that the principal centres of research were at medical schools, most notably at Toronto and McGill. He was impressed that outstanding research was being carried out by Collip and Selye at McGill and by Wilder Penfield at the Montreal Neurological Institute. He also made note of the work of A.T. Cameron and Bruce Chown at the University of Manitoba.

Banting remarked that a promising number of more junior investigators across the country displayed an interest in research but were hampered by their huge teaching loads and the shortage of funds for technical assistance and equipment. This type of situation was certainly one with which Collip was familiar, recalling his early days in Edmonton. Banting and Stewart concluded that there was a great need for funds to encourage students to take up research training. Banting noted, for example, that the University of Alberta medical school was more fortunate than many others he had visited because it had a larger number of full-time professional members on staff – three each in the departments of anatomy, bacteriology, biochemistry, and physiology and two in pathology. Laboratory space and other facilities were very good, and those in the Department of Biochemistry were outstanding (probably as a result of Collip's tenure there). However, a number of the faculty mentioned that their greatest need was the provision of scholarships and bursaries to keep promising students in research work. The few students who were engaged in research had to pay for their own supplies and equipment on top of paying tuition.

Collip had experienced regional disparities in the course of his career, having worked at the top two centres of medical research in Canada but also at a struggling, young institution. These differences emerged as a theme in Banting's survey. Because of the lack of funds and facilities, the vast majority of graduates of Maritime and western Canadian universities had to leave for post-graduate training in Toronto and Montreal or in the United States and Britain. After their training was complete, few returned to the Maritimes or the West because not many academic posts were available. Researchers in these regions experienced intellectual isolation from others working in their fields; they suggested that travelling fellowships would be helpful in overcoming this difficulty. Collip had of course been preoccupied with the expense of travel while at Alberta.

Banting also gained some support for the idea of establishing a research journal. Two medical journals existed at that time, the *Canadian Journal of Public Health*, founded in 1910, and the *Canadian Medical Association Journal*, founded in 1911. Both emphasized subjects more closely related to clinical practice than to investigation.

Banting's Canada-wide consultation may have stimulated interest in research among students and faculty across the country. G.H. Ettinger, a member of the first Associate Committee, commented that "in the small centres, particularly, he was welcomed almost as a Messiah; tired teachers had their hopes for assistance reawakened; young men and women became ardent disciples."[16]

The budget of the Associate Committee was $53,000 for its first year, $25,000 of which was committed to the research program in tuberculosis. The remainder was distributed as small grants-in-aid to researchers who had submitted requests for assistance. The response in the first year was great, with requests for over $125,000. Banting wrote to Penfield: "There has thus been an awakening on the part of research workers which we must do our best to assist."[17]

The pattern of providing extramural support for university research rather than establishing central laboratories was set early on in the work of the committee, more by default than by deliberate policy. The committee had quite a modest budget, and given this fact, its members acted on McNaughton's suggestion that they "should first endeavour to make the best use of existing facilities." A.G. Fleming, dean of medicine at McGill, agreed that this approach was in keeping with the will of representatives at the organizational meeting: "The feeling of the Conference was for men rather than for bricks and mortar." This practice contrasted with the model set by the British Medical Research Council, which employed staff at a central research institution and at its research units at medical schools. The Americans also had an extensive intramural program of research at the National Institutes of Health.[18]

The plans for the committee were interrupted the following year with the outbreak of war. More than in any previous conflict, science assumed a central position in all aspects of warfare. The NRC became the focus of scientific activities to support the war effort in Canada. The staff and budget of the council increased enormously within months of the outbreak of hostilities. By 1943 the budget was five times its prewar size.[19]

The medical research arm was dramatically changed as well. The Associate Committee placed its services at the disposal of the government and acted to investigate and advise on research problems related to the health of military and civilian populations. By 1942 much of the peace-time research program of the committee had been suspended in favour of work to support the war effort. At university laboratories across the country, fundamental research and most graduate training was put aside.

Three additional associate committees were created, one to deal with medical research in each of the three branches of the armed services. Banting, Best, and Collip, the surviving members of the insulin team, served as leaders of Canadian medical research. Each was associated with one of the wartime committees. Banting chaired the Committee on Aviation Medical Research, and he and his department at Toronto were heavily involved in studies in this area. Best entered the naval service and was named chair of the Naval Medical Research Associate Committee; during the war, he carried out research on seasickness. Collip was attached to the Army Medical Research Associate Committee. If there was any continued animosity among the three men, their separate roles and responsibilities no doubt helped to avert any problems.[20]

In September 1939 Collip was made vice-chairman of the main medical research committee under Banting, and he took over meetings during Banting's frequent absences. Banting and I.M. Rabinowitch visited Britain in December and January to establish a liaison with the British Medical Research Council in its war work. The British initially underestimated the research capabilities of the Canadian scientific community, but the Canadians gradually demonstrated their ability to contribute to the Allied cause and to carry out work on important projects independently.

Banting's special interest was in aviation medicine, and he and his associates explored problems experienced by airmen. William Franks, of Banting's laboratory, developed the first anti-g suit to allow pilots to withstand the high gravity forces they faced in dives and turns without blacking out. Banting was also very concerned with the threat of bacteriological warfare. Although he could not persuade the British medical research establishment to share his concern, he pushed for Canadian research on this subject. He created the top-secret committee (later the M-1000 Committee) that investigated ways of spreading disease organisms such as plague, cholera, anthrax, rabies, and typhus to human and animal populations.[21]

Upon Banting's death in February 1941, Collip assumed the chair of the Associate Committee on Medical Research with Harold Ettinger as his honorary secretary. Collip's responsibilities were considerable, since he was not only the chairman of the central coordinating committee but also an ex-officio member of the three wartime associate committees. Collip's daughter Barbara recalls that he was always very anxious about maintaining the secrecy of the many files he had to study, worrying when domestic help or even friends of his children came to the house. Barr and Rossiter observe, "Collip more than any other man had responsibilities for and knowledge of the entire spectrum of medical research carried out in Canada during World War II."[22]

Collip's duties increased even further when he was appointed medical liaison officer to the United States. For this purpose, he was made acting lieutenant-colonel in the Royal Canadian Army Medical Corps in 1942 and promoted to acting colonel in 1944. The liaison work required him to travel extensively and left him little time in Montreal. Abe Neufeld also left the laboratory to serve as a resident liaison officer in Washington.[23]

The three associate committees delegated a number of important wartime projects to subcommittees. One subcommittee was created to investigate the problems of infections. E.G.D. Murray of McGill, Philip H. Greey of Toronto, and Guilford B. Reed of Queen's contributed studies on such subjects as gas gangrene and the use of sulphonamides in the treatment of infections. In May 1941 Howard Florey of Oxford visited North America, meeting with Collip at McGill and Greey in Toronto to establish arrangements for the large-scale production of penicillin, probably the most important medical development of the war. Greey and Colin C. Lucas of Toronto initiated a pilot plant for the production of penicillin. The director general of the Army Medical Services furnished the funds so that the Connaught Laboratory could remodel a section of the Knox College building at the University of Toronto to serve as a centre for manufacture. Ayerst, McKenna and Harrison in Montreal was also invited to participate, and later a third firm was added, so that by the end of the war, Canadian companies were producing 20 billion units of penicillin a month, enough to meet all Canadian needs.[24]

A subcommittee on shock and blood substitutes involved researchers at Toronto and McGill. Collip and Denstedt explored the preservation of whole blood, while Best's group at Toronto experimented with methods of preparing dried blood serum. Collip, Noble, Selye, and J.S.L. Browne at McGill and R.A Cleghorn at the Banting Institute investigated the relation of shock to the adrenal cortex. This area of research attracted a great deal of attention because of the hope held by investigators that adrenocortical hormones could help pilots deal with shock and fatigue. Additional impetus was given by a secret report that suggested that the enemy was giving top priority to studying the use of adrenal hormones in commando training. The Canadian researchers concluded, however, that cortical extracts could not prevent or alleviate shock. In the United States, Edward Kendall had prepared small quantities of several different cortical extracts by the mid-1930s. Although the war focused scientific attention on these compounds, interest waned when it seemed that one of them (Compound A) was ineffective in treating shock. Nevertheless, Kendall persisted in trying to reproduce the closely related Compound E, even though there was little clinical interest in it. The therapeutic value of the drug was established after the war in 1949, when Philip Hench demonstrated that Compound E (cortisone) was useful in treating rheumatoid arthritis.[25]

Wilder Penfield chaired a third subcommittee – on surgery – that set up regional groups at McGill and the University of Montreal, Toronto, London, and Winnipeg. Surgical specialists conducted research on thermal burns, orthopaedic surgery, traumatic injuries of the nervous system, radiology, plastic surgery, and wound infections.

A fourth subcommittee dealt with the industrial health problems created on the home front. These investigators examined the physiological and psychological problems of fatigue and inadequate nutrition especially in the women who had moved into the war plants. Studies were also made of nutrition in civilian and military populations.[26]

After Banting's death, Collip reconstituted the committee on bacteriological warfare under the chairmanship of E.G.D. Murray. Murray, Guilford Reed, and Charles Mitchell of the Department of Agriculture were active in studying bacteriological weapons from both a defensive and an offensive perspective. The M-1000 Committee established a plant for the mass production of anthrax on Grosse-Ile in the St Lawrence. The Canadian project was abandoned later when the Americans developed the capability of producing anthrax in a safer and more efficient manner. Some medical scientists, such as Philip Greey, were uneasy about being involved in bacteriological warfare. Greey was more prepared to throw himself into the work on the production of penicillin. Others, however, were confident that studying and producing biological weapons was an appropriate response to a real wartime threat.[27]

NRC president C.J. Mackenzie remembered:

Some may differ, but I would not have thought of Collip as primarily a good conventional administrator. I don't think he would have made an outstanding President of a University or a Corporation for, as you know, his mind worked very fast and because he was impatient he never developed the art of patient-exposition; he was always miles ahead of his words and the current discussion.

He was not particularly articulate in formal meetings but, nevertheless, in my opinion (and I used to attend most medical meetings at N.R.C. during the war out of genuine interest) he was a good chairman. He was always courteous, fair and rarely showed the impatience I often thought he felt.

In my opinion the key to Collip's success in his role as head of N.R.C.'s medical activities was his pre-eminent scientific talents and standing as a research scientist. His reputation as a medical scientist not only made his task as chairman of committees easier, but of greater and, to me, of prime importance his knowledge and devotion to all medical research meant that he knew all the research workers in Canada and had a sound appreciation of the quality of their work. This meant that when the rapid expansion of war work was taking place Collip knew who were the proper men to head the innumerable research groups that were being set up and as chairman he had the power to have them so placed.

If one of the essential tests of a good administrator is the insight to select the best men for the key positions involved and then give them responsibility with only the most general review of objectives reached, then Collip's contribution as an administrator during the war must be rated high.[28]

The war had turned investigators' attention away from fundamental research to a narrow range of practical problems. The emergency situation also forced a close collaboration and coordination among academic researchers and industrial scientists. The mass production of penicillin was one major achievement that emerged from this intense, cooperative atmosphere. Yet, while key developments in some fields were accelerated, many other fields lay neglected. As was the case with Collip, it could prove difficult for researchers to pick up the pieces of peacetime research programs when the war came to a close.

The legacy of the wartime committees was the creation of a permanent institutional structure for the funding and coordination of medical research in Canada. The war had provided an opportunity for proponents of research to demonstrate the utility of medical science and to demand a great increase in funding. Also, a great number of junior personnel had been brought into scientific work through war research projects; many of them remained on after the war. Some 120 scientific publications were supported by grants made between 1938 and 1946. At the close of the war, the Associate Committee members sought to consolidate these gains by arguing that the same sum that had been spent by all four medical research associate committees during the war would be required for post war activities. One of the tasks they faced was to place personnel returning from military service. At the urging of Wilder Penfield, the Associate Committee on Medical Research initiated a system of graduate fellowships to provide research opportunities for medical officers returning to civilian life.[29]

The committee also took up P.H.T. Thorlackson's recommendation that a western regional group be established to stimulate research in the four western provinces. At these annual meetings, the researchers from the four western universities – British Columbia, Alberta, Saskatchewan, and Manitoba – gathered at one of their institutions to see one another's laboratories and to present papers in an informal setting. This helped to alleviate the problems of isolation experienced by the westerners and saved the expense of travelling to larger centres in central Canada. Collip and Ettinger travelled out to the first meeting, bringing a bit of the East to the West. Collip's interest in the West had endured since his days in Edmonton, and he was a strong supporter of these initiatives.[30]

At this juncture, the committee seriously debated the question of establishing an independent medical research council. One of the chief concerns was that a separate medical research council would likely be made responsible to an existing ministry of the federal government rather than to a committee of the cabinet, as was the NRC. After considerable discussion, the committee opted instead for the more cautious approach of gradual evolution within the NRC. The Associate Committee became the more autonomous Division of Medical Research, taking it one step closer to its goal of independence.[31]

THE DIVISION OF MEDICAL RESEARCH

Collip was made the first director of the new division, and his friend Harold Ettinger was made assistant director. The division started its work in 1946 with a budget of $200,000, almost a fourfold increase over the budget of the Associate Committee when it started in 1938. The Division of Medical Research differed from other divisions in the NRC in that its program was entirely extramural; no central laboratories were built. Throughout his tenure, Collip strongly opposed the establishment of a central research facility, choosing instead to vigorously extend the program of grants and fellowships to researchers at existing institutions.[32]

In 1948 the Privy Council commissioned a second national survey, conducted again by Chester Stewart, this time with Morley Whillans of the Defence Research Board and Ralph MacAulay of the Department of National Health and Welfare. In the ten years since the last survey, there had been a sizable increase in the number of junior faculty. The many new investigators who had been brought into medical research through wartime work had contributed their numbers to a rapid postwar expansion of the field. In its report, the Privy Council's committee noted that it could now count 955 persons in medical research at universities: 278 technicians, 315 graduate students, and 311 part-time and 51 full-time researchers. The committee also found an increased enthusiasm for research among those it surveyed, despite the continuing problems of a shortage of funds, crowded conditions, and heavy teaching loads. Stewart and his colleagues noted that, as before, most research was being conducted in medical schools, university departments, and special institutes. Some research work was also carried out in pharmaceutical houses, hospitals, and institutions apart from medical schools, in provincial and federal health laboratories, and by the Department of National Defence. The growing body of Canadian scientific studies had also warranted the creation of new research journals. The *Revue Canadienne de Biologie* had been established in 1942. Through the work of the Associate Committee on Medical Research, the NRC also authorized a medical research section in the *Canadian Journal of Research* (section E) in 1944. Collip served as the editor of this journal and of its successors – the *Canadian Journal of Medical Sciences* (1951–53) and the *Canadian Journal of Biochemistry and Physiology* (1954–56) – for a total of twelve years.[33]

The report identified three especially pressing needs: (1) senior research appointments that would provide positions for those who might otherwise have to go into clinical practice or to other countries; (2) the assurance of continuity in research; and (3) easier methods of administering grants. To meet these needs, the division developed an expanded program of extramural grants to university scientists. These grants were used to stimulate research, provide for travel opportunities, create university appointments, and train young graduates.

The Division of Medical Research of the 1950s was much less interventionist than Banting might have envisioned it being in 1938. The advisory committee chose not to direct resources to particular research problems; instead it selected projects from the applications submitted by interested investigators. The fellowship program was aimed at assisting ex-servicemen who sought graduate training to prepare for the examinations of the Royal College of Physicians and Surgeons. Senior research fellowships were created for graduates in medicine who were preparing for careers in research. By 1954, serious concern arose about the pressing need to provide talented young investigators with the opportunity to devote themselves entirely to research. The senior research fellowships were replaced in 1955 by medical research associateships, that served to establish university appointments for medical scientists with salaries like those of the research officers at NRC institutions. The universities provided the appointments, while the NRC paid the salaries for these associates.[34]

The division members further acknowledged the growing trend towards collaborative research by instituting a new type of award known as the "consolidated grant." This grant was made to a laboratory group as a whole rather than being split into a number of grants-in-aid to individuals. The consolidated grant provided easier administration as well as longer-term support than had been previously available. Collip certainly felt the need for this type of grant in his own case. As the head of a large group of researchers at the University of Western Ontario, he was quite apprehensive about building up the department, often fearful for the security of his associates if funding were to be cut. Collip was among the first recipients of these grants, along with Best, Penfield, and J.S.L. Browne.[35]

NEW SOURCES OF RESEARCH FUNDING

As before, medical research had a base of support in general university funds, but during this period, in addition to the NRC's Division of Medical Research, a number of other new sources became available. During the postwar years, several voluntary societies for the study of special diseases were formed, notably the National Cancer Institute and the Canadian Arthritis and Rheumatism Society. They and philanthropic foundations, pharmaceutical firms, and private gifts brought additional funds to research.

An interesting case of a privately funded research institution was the W.P. Caven Research Foundation (1949–1974), one of Canada's first independent research facilities. This small clinical research laboratory, created for Toronto surgeon Dr Gordon Murray by his supporters, ultimately failed in its attempt to cultivate medical research outside an academic setting. Shelley McKellar argues than the foundation, lacking the status and resources of a university setting, had difficulty attracting high-calibre researchers. Moreover, Murray failed to participate in the system of grantsmanship that was becoming the norm during this period, coming, as he did, from a generation of investigators who expected to receive support for their professional standing or past accomplishments rather than their ability to write detailed research proposals and reports.[36]

Apart from through the Division of Medical Research, governmental support was also channelled through the Defence Research Board and the Department of National Health and Welfare. In 1948 the federal government instituted Public Health Grants to support research in the field of public health. In order to coordinate the activities of these many granting agencies, ad hoc conferences were held to review applications and determine the appropriate body to which they should be routed. The Division of Medical Research took a coordinating role in these activities, aiding the National Cancer Institute and the Canadian

Arthritis and Rheumatism Society by reviewing and making recommendations on their applications for research grants and fellowships.[37]

NRC president E.W.C. Steacie, who took office in 1952, was himself an academic chemist and a strong advocate of basic research. Furthermore, he held the conviction that fundamental work was best carried out primarily at universities. While there was a strong rivalry between the medical arm of the NRC and the other governmental bodies that supported medical research, these agencies gradually began to differentiate their roles. Collip displayed his own bias towards basic research when he argued, "Personally, I am in favour of an expansion of clinical research by competent workers, but if our funds are to be limited I feel sure that we will get the best value for the money expended if we use most, if not all of it, in supporting fundamental work in the basic medical sciences."[38] Over time, the NRC medical research division moved towards the support of fundamental research, while the Department of Veterans Affairs and the Public Health Research Fund supplied funds for clinical studies in such fields as psychiatry, obstetrics, paediatrics, and epidemiology.[39]

Chester Stewart notes that there was considerable competition for federal funds between the NRC's Division of Medical Research and the Department of Health and Welfare's national health research grants. During the 1950s the national health grants grew at an unprecedented rate, and Stewart argues that this was "particularly galling to the pre-clinical scientists."[40] By 1955 these grants had a budget of $1,785,000, more than a million dollars greater than that of the NRC division.[41]

DEVELOPING RESEARCH ON A NATIONAL BASIS

The idea of an independent medical research council continued to be debated through these years. Ray Farquharson of the University of Toronto discussed the idea with Steacie in 1954. As before, political questions about funds and authority continued to be obstacles. Farquharson reported to Collip:

We talked about the possibility of developing a separate Medical Research Council for which so many of our colleagues are now pressing, thinking that it would have disposal of all the federal funds for medical research. The President confirms my fears that it would be difficult to acquire the large sums now disposed of by the Department of Health and Welfare and, further, that a Medical Research Council would almost certainly have to report to the Minister of Health and Welfare. It could hardly be hoped that a Medical Research Council would be so fortunate as to be left to develop its policies without political pressure. I think that it is much better for medical research to continue to build as part of the National Research Council.[42]

Another part of the division's work was the distribution of hormone products that were available only in limited quantities. After Philip Hench and Edward Kendall reported the effect of cortisone on rheumatoid arthritis in 1949, many scientists were eager to explore cortisone's effects on this and other diseases. This interest extended to adrenocorticotrophic hormone (ACTH), the pituitary hormone that stimulates the adrenal glands to produce cortisone. This project was particularly close to Collip's heart, since he was the one who had successfully produced the first active preparation of ACTH years before. The division oversaw the Canadian production and distribution of cortisone and ACTH for research purposes. After 1953, the division also coordinated the supply of growth hormone.[43]

The members of the Division of Medical Research had to deal with the difficult question of whether to channel support to institutions that were already well established or to distribute the funds more widely and promote the growth of new research centres. Here, practice rather than explicit policy became important. Ettinger and Collip worked closely in evaluating the applications as they came in. Ettinger would compare the referees' reports against the money available in the budget and adjust the prospective grants to fit. Years later, Chester Stewart praised these early officers for having "the wisdom to deviate from their own rules" by encouraging beginners and strengthening weak departments. He noted, for example, that officers provided such "special treatment" and "leniency" as sending constructive comments on grant applications and allowing applicants the opportunity to revise their proposals. Stewart argues that these actions allowed medical research to develop on a national basis rather than only at those institutions that were already strong.[44]

Collip attracted some criticism for not pushing hard enough to strengthen the division's position. His colleagues Ettinger and Noble speculate that he may have been too timid about trying to raise the division's budget. They suggest that this may have been because Collip had personal difficulties in working with the NRC presidents, C.J. Mackenzie, who they say "had the ability to overwhelm" him, and "Ned" Steacie, who they believe Collip felt was hostile to him. This lack of assertiveness seems surprising in light of Collip's forceful and successful campaigns for financial compensation in his own academic career.[45]

In 1957 the Division of Medical Research reached the final stage of its separation from the NRC. Collip had favoured the creation of an independent medical research council, but this was not to happen during his tenure. That year, at the age of sixty-five, he retired from the directorship and was succeeded by Ray Farquharson. The initiative for the move to full independence came from the Association of Canadian Medical Colleges, which was made up of the deans of the medical schools. They expressed the concern that the federal funds available for research were insufficient to meet the requirements of a field that was now rapidly growing. Ettinger stated the case strongly: "There is a great unrest in the medical research laboratories of universities because it is believed that this total sum ($5,535,000) is inadequate and that the multiplicity of sources makes administration awkward and continuity uncertain."[46]

A number of factors contributed to the greatly increased need for research support. First, there had been a sudden expansion of scientific programs in the universities in the postwar period. Second, two new medical schools had been established, the first at the University of Ottawa and the second at the University of British Columbia. The program at the University of Saskatchewan had also been expanded to four years. The nature of research was changing, too, requiring more expensive research equipment and more extensive facilities. Finally, there had been a great expansion in the scope of medical science itself. The deans resolved to ask the prime minister to increase the funds by at least $500,000.

A third study was commissioned at this time. Ray Farquharson headed up the Special Committee to Review the Extramural Support of Medical Research. The committee collected and evaluated written submissions by and interviews with representatives of all Canadian institutions associated with medical research. As well, it gathered comparative statements from the United States, the United Kingdom, Australia, and Sweden. NRC medical research support amounted to almost one and a half million dollars, and the Department of National Health and Welfare and the Defence Research Board added another two and a half million. (This figure does not include the general university funds provided by the provincial governments.) In comparison, the U.S. National Institutes of Health spent $108 million on medical research, or approximately twice as much as a percentage of its gross national product. The review committee concluded that funding had not kept pace with the growth in research. It found grave inadequacies in the grants and fellowships programs, in the salaries of scientific staff, in fluid funds in medical schools, and in the construction of research facilities. The committee recommended that longer-term grants be made to ensure continuity of research and that greater flexibility be permitted in the use of funds to allow researchers to pursue long-term goals.[47]

The Farquharson committee commended the NRC division's decision to channel its resources through the universities and teaching hospitals rather than to establish central laboratories. It argued that medical research is unique in that it requires a close association with medical schools to reach its full development. The committee also regarded this association as crucial for the recruitment and training of young investigators and for stimulating teaching.[48]

As had been originally planned, the medical research arm of the NRC had been gaining increased funding and autonomy within the council over the twenty years since its inception. The Farquharson committee concluded that this development was now complete: "The time has come to take the final step and establish an independent Medical Research Council. This opinion is shared by virtually all medical research workers in Canada, and those consulted in other countries."[49]

The review committee argued that Canadian medical research had grown tremendously and that it should now be directed by a body directly reporting to the Privy Council through its Committee on Scientific and Industrial Research rather than through a department of government. In 1960 the Medical Research Council of Canada (MRC) was established. The transition, however, was complicated by a change in government, and the final legislation was not passed until 1968. Thus, for several years the MRC remained within the orbit of the NRC and obtained its funding through joint grants.

LAYING THE FOUNDATIONS

The policies and practices established by the Associate Committee and the Division of Medical Research assisted the growth of medical research and shaped its institutions in the postwar period. Change was brought about through a cautious, evolutionary approach. The division consolidated the gains achieved by the wartime associate committees and was effective in using these advances to meet the gravest needs of the research enterprise – the funding of established researchers, the training of students, the provision of travel grants, and the establishment of academic posts. Because of financial constraints and the relatively small size of the research community in Canada, the program of the Associate Committee and Division of Medical Research was entirely extramural. Funds were channelled to universities and teaching hospitals to help create a system in which medical research was closely tied with medical education. The Associate Committee and the division also promoted the growth of research on a truly national basis. They actively developed policies and practices that stimulated research not only in the established centres but also across the country. As head of the NRC's medical research arm for sixteen years, Collip brought his own experience, as well as his own sympathies, to bear on the development of research policy. As one of the few who had been able to succeed in the period of private funding, he was well placed to guide Canadian medical research into a new era of government support and coordination.

C.J. MacKenzie would later evaluate Collip's contribution:

While Collip's outstanding talent undoubtedly lay in the field of fundamental research I think his leadership in the field of organized support of medical research during those 19 years should not be minimized, as it was in the war and post war years that the foundations were layed [sic] for the sane, rapid and admirable way in which large scale medical research has developed in Canada.

Of course Collip was not wholly responsible as the growth was influenced by the active contribution of a substantial number of medical workers, including people like Banting, Duncan Graham, Best, Hurst Brown, Ettinger and Farquharson who headed research organizations of N.R.C. in war and peace, as well as by scores of research men and officers in universities, other departments and organizations, but after all Collip was the active director of N.R.C. medical research during those formative years and 19 years of successful building is a monument to any director.[50]

8

Dean of Medicine, 1947–1965

It seems in retrospect he was always arriving or departing, always in a hurry.[1]
C.J. Mackenzie to F.G. MacIntosh, 19 October 1965

Collip spent the remainder of his career in London as dean of medicine at the University of Western Ontario.[2] The postwar period was a time of active expansion in the medical school at Western, just as it was at other medical schools across the country. The size of the medical class grew, as did the number of graduate students. An honours course in the basic medical sciences was instituted. Collip oversaw the expansion in facilities and led the medical school in its move from its old location across town to the main university campus. Collip was still active, restless, and straining against limits. As always, he moved abruptly and spoke quickly, and he was notorious for speeding through campus and leaving his car wherever he wanted. The grounds staff soon learned to recognize the dean's car and were under instruction not to ticket it. The medical students developed a shorthand method to indicate the presence of the dean in their annual comedy revue – a spray of gravel dashed against a wall.

For Ray and Bert, life changed quite dramatically. Their home life in Montreal had been relatively quiet, especially during the war years when Collip had been busy travelling on official business and so concerned about keeping national secrets that he rarely had people to the house. They were now responsible for hosting many visitors, and they opened their home to the medical class every year. Ray was well known for the warmth and graciousness with which she welcomed guests to the many catered functions she was expected to hold as the wife of the dean. Together, they basked in the company of the young students and enjoyed taking an interest in their lives. To the surprise of Collip's friends and perhaps even his family, he took to administrative work wholeheartedly, relishing the idea of leading the development of the medical school. When asked about his administrative skills, though, tactful friends respond that Collip was never very keen on the details but was always blessed with good assistants. It was not always easy dealing with the inevitable jealousies and animosities between different factions within the medical school and within the larger community. A.C. Wallace, a pathologist and researcher in Collip's lab, recalls Collip telling him that he sometimes found this sort of thing difficult to take, but that he regarded these challenges as something he had to beat.[3]

In addition to running the medical school as a whole, he was head of the Department of Medical Research. The department was housed in a building originally intended for the Department of Zoology. Bob Noble, several graduate students (including Ken Carroll, Kay Maclean, and Burwell Taylor), three technicians (Hans Pedersen, Axel Andersen, and Rheinhold Rasmussen), and his long-time loyal assistant Arthur Long from Edmonton days had followed Collip from McGill. Collip's old friend the bacteriologist E.G.D. "Joburg" Murray joined the department after his retirement from McGill. In 1960 Collip was able to lure another old friend, Abe Neufeld, to Western as well. Other staff, J.A.F. Stevenson, R.W. Begg, and Charles Engle, were brought into the department, too. When Collip and his staff arrived in 1947, another storey and a wing were added to accommodate them. The building was named the Collip Medical Research Laboratory.

On a typical day, Collip would spend the morning at the dean's office looking after his duties there, but after lunch, he would spend his time in the laboratory. He remained very interested in the activities of his junior associates. Although, he was now clearly a world-renowned figure in medical research, even young researchers were struck by the fact that he did not seem to have the polish or the aloofness they might have expected. They found him sincere in his speech, natural – he was not one to put on airs – perhaps even somewhat awkward, but eminently approachable. Wallace recalls that Collip would often be sitting in his office with his door open, reading a few articles – and he could read at a ferocious rate – but that he would put everything down to listen to whatever problems were brought to him. And he could often solve the problem, too, because he knew how to attack the question, where to find more information, or how to get more money or equipment. He sometimes astounded his staff and students with his grasp of the current literature, and he did everything he could to make it possible for them to pursue their ideas. Robert Macbeth remembers Collip as being at his best on such occasions; when he discussed a research problem one-on-one, he became very animated, very much alive. However, Collip never found his way back to the bench himself. For quite some time, he continued to say he might like to get back to making his extracts. He never did. For years, the faithful Arthur Long kept his chief's equipment polished and ready for his return, guarding it fiercely even when everyone else in the lab was running out of glassware. A monstrous new German Palder still, with a tremendous capacity for extracting huge amounts of material, was especially installed for Collip, but stood unused.[4]

Now that Collip was often busy with his work in the dean's office, it was left to Bob Noble to set the tone for the laboratory. Noble's easygoing, jovial style made the lab a more relaxed place than it had been in its heyday at McGill. Gone was the ethos that had kept the Montreal lab humming until late into the night. Ken Carroll recalls that it sometimes seemed as though the lab at Western started planning for its Christmas party as early as August and that plenty of effort would be devoted to organizing skits and such things. This did not mean that the work of the group was not stimulating and important. Endocrinology continued to be central to the work of the lab group, but they extended their interests to atherosclerosis, cancer, and synthetic steroids. In 1957 Bob Noble and chemist Charles Beer isolated an alkaloid product from the periwinkle plant that they named "vincaleucoblastine" (or "vinblastine"). This turned out to be a most important achievement. Vinblastine was found to be a valuable treatment for leukaemia and Hodgkin's disease, and grew to become one of the most commonly used cancer chemotherapy drugs.[5]

ELDER STATESMAN

Throughout his career, Collip took a leading role in the development of medical research as a profession. As dean of medicine, he was a member of the Association of Canadian Medical Colleges, and he served as president for one term. He guided the development of the National Research Council's *Canadian Journal of Research*, Section E, in 1944, the first Canadian research journal for medical sciences. Collip edited it and its successors until 1956. He was the first president (1936) of the Canadian Physiological Society and was the only member to serve a second term as president (1952). He was also one of the early presidents of the American Association for the Study of Internal Secretions (1925–26), counsellor of the American Society of Biological Chemists (1937), and a delegate to the League of Nations Committee on Standardization of Hormones during the 1930s.

Collip's achievements were recognized in later years with many honours and awards. He received the Order of the British Empire (1943)

and the U.S. Medal of Freedom with Silver Palm (1947) for his war efforts. He was made a Fellow of the Royal Society of Canada (1925)
and subsequently became the society's president (1942–43). He was
also elected as Fellow of the Royal Society of London (1933). He was
awarded fellowships in several clinical societies as well: the American
College of Physicians (1930), the Royal College of Physicians of Canada (1931), the Royal College of Physicians of London (1938), and the
American College of Obstetricians and Gynecologists (1947). In 1936
he received the Flavelle Medal of the Royal Society of Canada and the
F.N.G. Starr Medal of the Canadian Medical Association; in 1937, the
Cameron Prize from the University of Edinburgh; in 1941, the Charles
Mickle Award of the University of Toronto; and in 1960, the Banting
Medal of the American Diabetes Association. He had twelve honorary
degrees conferred upon him by universities in Canada, Britain, and the
United States. On his sixty-fifth birthday, his friends, colleagues, and
former students prepared a special issue of the *Canadian Journal of
Biochemistry and Physiology* in his honour. Efforts were made by
friends at McGill and the University of Western Ontario to secure a
Nobel Prize for him, but without success.

Collip was now an elder statesman of medical research, but the restless personality and drive that had brought him this far meant he could
never be "retiring." When he reached the age of sixty-five, Collip faced
mandatory retirement from his work at the National Research Council.
His daughter Barbara and Robert Noble remember the forced retirement as something he took very hard. Barbara Wyatt says, "It broke
him." Noble and Harold Ettinger suggest that there was some incompatibility between Collip and NRC president Steacie and that Collip
was hurt at the way the retirement was handled. Collip remained dean
at Western for two more years, stepping down in 1961. He retained his
position as head of the medical research department, however, and continued to look in on the work there, though by this time Robert Noble
had gone on to the University of British Columbia, where he had been
offered the opportunity to head up his own laboratory in cancer research. Collip's daughter and son-in-law recall that he seemed never
really happy again after having to retire.[6]

Still, Collip had the abiding support and companionship of his wife,
and he could enjoy watching his children start families of their own.
Margaret had recovered from the worst of her Grave's disease and had
gone on to marry Gerald McBride. Barbara had studied medicine at
McGill and then did a master's in endocrinology there as well. This
meant that she had to work in her father's lab and even had to take her
oral examination with her father and Bob Noble. During her studies,
she had met Jackson Wyatt, a clinician from the American South who

was doing his residency at the Royal Victoria Hospital. They married and moved to Rome, Georgia, where Barbara practised in geriatric medicine. The Collip's youngest child, Jack, also studied medicine. He married and settled in Edmonton practising anaesthesia.

In retirement, Bert and Ray Collip continued to be inseparable, receiving visits from their children and many grandchildren – Margaret's five, Barbara's five, and Jack's four (of which one was born only after Bert Collip's death). They loved making impromptu journeys as well. On one trip, they telegraphed Barbara and C.J. Wyatt from Chattanooga, announcing only "We'll be there in an hour." In June 1965 Bert and Ray made another one of their famous cross-country drives to attend the meeting of the Royal Society in Vancouver. On the way, they stopped in Edmonton to visit with their son, Jack. In Vancouver, they met with long-time friend Bob Noble and his wife. The Collips drove back east, putting their car on the ferry at Thunder Bay and returning safely to London. Two days later, Bert Collip suffered a stroke. In his later years, he had grown more stout and had developed dangerously high blood pressure. He was admitted to the university hospital, where he died quietly, at the age of seventy-two.

Collip's funeral was an august affair with a hundred honorary pallbearers from all over Canada and the United States. Ray, his constant companion in life, bravely faced the funeral and a large reception at her home. Later in the evening, she stoically watched the broadcast of the burial ceremony on television. Tributes poured in from colleagues and friends everywhere, celebrating her husband's remarkable achievements.

Conclusion:
The Transformation
of the Research Enterprise

In the early decades of the twentieth century, medical research in Canada was the pursuit of an exceptional few. By mid-century, it had burgeoned into a systematic, large-scale enterprise involving teams of professional scientists and dozens of laboratories in universities, government, and industry. J.B. Collip – driven, devoted, and marvellously skilled in drawing biological gold from dross – was a noteworthy part of this change. His story gives us some insight into the forces that transformed the landscape of Canadian medical research.

Collip's life and scientific work stretched across a key period in the development of medical research in Canada. His career was an exceptional one, and yet his varied experiences of scientific life reflect many facets of Canadian medical research during its formative years.

Yves Gingras developed an analytic model to study the formation of scientific communities and has applied it to the development of physics, the first scientific community to be constituted in Canada. The first phase he identifies is the emergence of research practice. The second is the institutionalization of research whereby structures are set up to allow the production of knowledge and the "reproduction" of the next generation of scientists. The final phase is the creation of a social identity through the establishment of research journals and scientific societies.[1]

In the Canadian medical research community, the first phase of this development was initiated by pioneers like Robert Ramsay Wright and A.B. Macallum, who created an honours stream in biochemistry and physiology that was dedicated to the pursuit of original investigation. These pioneers produced Collip's generation of investigators – those of the second phase – who were firmly imbued with the research ideal and fully expected that research was to be a component of their academic careers. This generation reshaped universities in its demand to secure institutional conditions that would favour research. The challenges that Collip faced characterized this stage of development: to set up the structures conducive to research and to train students. The final phase of development, the creation of a social identity, began with the creation of the Canadian Physiological Society in 1934–35, was nurtured by the creation of a Canadian research journal for medical science in 1944, but only fully flowered in the 1950s with the creation of the Canadian Federation of Biological Societies, a group that included biochemical, physiological, anatomical, and pharmacological scientists.

As a student of research pioneer Macallum, Collip was privileged to have his undergraduate and graduate education at the one university in Canada where he could get rigorous training in original research in biochemistry. He was among the early group of Canadians able to earn a PhD in this country. Because of the expansion of existing universities and the creation of new universities in the West, scientists of his generation were able to acquire academic posts in Canada; there was no longer the need to travel to the United States or abroad as most others had before. Even so, Collip was one of only three PhDs that Macallum produced, and most of his colleagues in Canadian university posts were trained elsewhere, the majority in Britain.

At the University of Alberta, Collip experienced the struggles of the new generation as it tried to eke out a place for research in academic posts that were geared towards teaching. Although he had the sympathy of a fellow scientist in his president, H.M. Tory, Collip continued to be restricted by the lack of research funds and by the teaching load that was demanded of him because of biochemistry's position as a service course in the medical faculty. He also experienced the intellectual isolation of scientists located far from the established centres of central Canada. Nevertheless, Collip managed to cultivate his research interests in general biochemistry and by 1921 had made an impressive start to his career.

The discovery of insulin was a turning point in Collip's career, as it was in the development of the medical research community in Canada. The discovery, and Collip's contribution to it, was a culmination of the work done by Ramsay Wright and Macallum in establishing a strong research tradition and developing excellent laboratory facilities at the University of Toronto.[2] The impact of the insulin discovery was significant. Banting, and to a lesser extent Best and Collip, became the focal point of Canadian pride. After Banting's death, Best and Collip took on the leadership in medical research. In the field of endocrinology, insulin marked an important breakthrough in establishing the legitimacy of a young field plagued by its associations with quackery. While Collip never received full public recognition for his role in the discovery during his lifetime, he benefited immensely from his association with the achievement. His share of the insulin royalties provided him with a large and long-term source of research funds that was unrivalled in Canada, save for Banting and Best. The prestige of his association with the work also drew other donations from private benefactors and philanthropic foundations. Before insulin, Collip was certainly one of the promising young medical researchers in the country. After insulin, his place as a leader in the field was secured.

Collip's role in the insulin discovery diverted his research career from its original path in general biochemistry to one in medical biochemistry, especially in the study of hormones with therapeutic value. While he took a broad approach to this field, his best-known achievements in subsequent years follow closely on the pattern set in the insulin work: the isolation and characterization of hormones useful in clinical therapy. His next major accomplishment, the preparation of an active extract of the parathyroid hormone, put him in the midst of a struggle by the fledgling profession of laboratory researchers to define themselves against traditional clinical styles of investigation in endocrine studies. His dispute with Hanson also reveals the challenges posed by the growing involvement of academic scientists in the commercial development of medical products. While collaborative ventures between pharmaceutical firms and academic researchers could benefit both parties, traditional codes regarding the creation and ownership of scientific knowledge were challenged.

At McGill, Collip became firmly established as a researcher. His place in McGill's faculty was part of the university's campaign to rebuild its leading position in medicine by cultivating fundamental and clinical research. The discovery of Emmenin and its subsequent commercial development fed into this plan by contributing a therapeutic product that was useful in both gaining public attention and generating new research funds. At McGill, Collip developed his talents as an entrepreneur of science, working to elaborate his post into a full-time research position and to nurture a growing group of students and associates. The conflict with the British Medical Research Council over the matter of patenting, with the result that Collip and McGill bowed to the MRC's demands, reveals the strong ties that English Canadian academics still had with Britain in matters of professional conduct. Nevertheless, the orientation of scientists like Collip was firmly turning to the United States, first because leadership in scientific research was passing to America during the 1920s and 1930s, and second, because the United States, through its large philanthropic foundations, was a principal source of research funds for Canadians.

During his "great years" at McGill, Collip was able to make the transition to the large-team collaborative style of research that was to become the dominant pattern in subsequent years. In doing this, he was in a small way part of a general trend in scientific research worldwide – moving from "little science" to "big science." He developed a broadly based research program that capitalized on the talents and disciplinary training of his associates. His greatest successes followed in the pattern of his insulin work because he excelled in manipulative biochemistry, especially in the extraction of active principles from glandular tissue. He was also fortunate to have a team of fine co-workers who then examined these extracts for their physiological activities. He and his group were on the forefront of endocrine research worldwide, and his many students, especially J.S.L. Browne, guaranteed that endocrinology would remain one of the principal areas in which Canadian medical scientists have made important contributions.

Collip's strengths and weaknesses are apparent. In the laboratory, his restless personality led him to make a long string of important contributions to science, but it also allowed him to take on too broad a research program, so that his energies were dissipated and results were sometimes rushed and not always thoroughly developed. As the director of a large group, he could be open to a wide variety of interests and yet intolerant of serious challenges to his research program. He could be benignly negligent and yet terribly demanding when a subject caught his fancy.

Collip succeeded in building a research group because he was an active entrepreneur of science. Finding funds for his laboratory was a time-consuming task and often fraught with failure. Learning from his experience with insulin, he actively sought the patenting and commercial development of any of his products with therapeutic potential. While some efforts failed – the parathyroid hormone for instance – others succeeded brilliantly, such as Emmenin and its successor, Premarin. The royalty funds accruing to him personally for use in research gave him an exceptional hand in his negotiations with his administrators. Collip actively sought funding from the Rockefeller Foundation but failed for scientific and administrative reasons. He was successful, however, in cultivating the acquaintance of prominent Canadians and attracting their donations.

His friends and students generally remember him as a shy, modest man, slow to his own defence yet bold in the support of others. This assessment contrasts sharply with the comments of his institutional superiors, who at times thought of him as ambitious, self-seeking, and

temperamental. As a person, he was quickly provoked by real or imag-
ined slights, especially when he felt that his accomplishments were not
adequately rewarded. As an institution builder, he had to wrestle with
his administrators to forge a secure place for his research endeavours.

His lifelong dream of a pure research post was finally fulfilled with
the creation of the Research Institute of Endocrinology, but ironically,
only when he was no longer able to use it. When he left McGill, the
Research Institute was quickly reabsorbed into the Department of
Biochemistry. Collip's institute did not set a trend for free-standing
institutes for fundamental medical research. Almost all basic medical
science remained tied to undergraduate teaching. The research department that was set up for Banting and later headed by Best remained
unique, a product of the insulin discovery.[3] The Department of Medical
Research set up for Collip at Western was terminated two years after
his death and, like his McGill institute, was reabsorbed back into
the traditional department structure. Thus, Collip's scientific legacy is
found not in the continuation of particular institutions but in the successful careers of his students and collaborators in many centres
throughout Canada and around the world.

Collip's varied experiences during his long career convinced him of
the need for systematic governmental support of medical research. He
recognized that his own position had been exceptional and that many
of his colleagues had far greater difficulty in conducting research and
recruiting students. A major barrier was the lack of funds. The involvement of medical investigators in the war effort carved a place for medical research in the public eye and in government funding structures.
Collip worked with the National Research Council during the war and
the boom of the postwar reconstruction period. The establishment of a
system of grants-in-aid, scholarships, and fellowships finally institutionalized medical research, making it more feasible for students to
pursue advanced studies and for senior investigators to make a career
of experimental work. As well as governmental funding, other sources
of support were developed at this time, such as the voluntary societies
and pharmaceutical firms.

Collip was also an active leader in the third phase of the development of the medical research community in Canada, the creation of a
social identity. He was a dominant figure in the guidance of the medical
research journal and in scientific and medical societies. His experiences
in many schools and regions of the country helped him to promote a
truly national vision of the research community.

Collip's story gains us insight into the rise of large-scale, systematic
government funding for medical research. For most of his career, Collip
had to piece together his research funds from a combination of public

and private sources. In doing so, he had to work through the implications of taking funds from private benefactors, public institutions, and corporations.

For scientists and their institutions today, the problem of navigating the scientific, ethical, and practical shoals of securing funding for research is more acute than ever, especially in relation to industry. In 2001, eighty years after the discovery of insulin and the start of the University of Toronto's relationship with Eli Lilly, the university faced a very public controversy. Psychiatrist David Healey accused the university of scuttling his appointment to a post at the Centre for Addiction and Mental Health (CAMH) and the Department of Psychiatry because of his critical remarks about Prozac, manufactured by Eli Lilly, the CAMH's largest sponsor. This led to a storm of media attention, with leading academics and media commentators expressing grave concern about the closeness of the relationship of industry to academia and about the challenge to academic freedom.[4] Nearby, at the University of Toronto teaching hospital the Hospital for Sick Children, Dr Nancy Olivieri was the focus of international attention when Apotex, the pharmaceutical company funding her clinical trials, attempted to suppress her findings of adverse side effects of its drug. A committee of inquiry noted, "The controversy arose in a context where public institutions now have to rely more on funding from private corporations, but haven't put in place adequate policies and practices to protect the public."[5]

In his day, Collip and his associates traversed this difficult terrain, negotiating issues as they arose, navigating through changing expectations and ethos, and hammering out pragmatic solutions that paved the way for the investigators and institutions of today. Collip was able to capitalize on his abilities, both as a talented researcher and an adept entrepreneur of science, to build an eventful and successful career for himself and to contribute to the institutionalization of medical research in Canada.

Notes

ABBREVIATIONS

CISTI Canadian Institute for Scientific and Technical Information
MUA McGill University Archives
NRC National Research Council
RAC Rockefeller Archive Center
RF Rockefeller Foundation
UAA University of Alberta Archives
UT University of Toronto
UTA University of Toronto Archives
UWO University of Western Ontario

INTRODUCTION

1 The most detailed biographical source on Collip is M.L. Barr and R.J. Rossiter, "James Bertram Collip, 1892–1965," *Biographical Memoirs of Fellows of the Royal Society* 19 (1973): 235–67.

2 Michael Bliss, *The Discovery of Insulin* (Toronto: McClelland and Stewart 1982). Bliss's view of Collip's neglected status is examined in Michael Bliss, "J.B. Collip: A Forgotten Member of the Insulin Team," in *Essays in the History of Canadian Medicine*, ed. Wendy Mitchinson and Janice P. Dickin McGinnis (Toronto: McClelland and Stewart 1988), 110–25.

CHAPTER ONE

1 J.B. Collip, "Addison Lecture, Guys Hospital," manuscript of a lecture never given, Collip Papers, MS Collection, 269, item 4, Fisher Rare Book Library, University of Toronto (hereafter UT).

2 *Directory of the County of Hastings* (Belleville, Ont., 1889); Nick Mika and Helma Mika, *Historic Belleville* (Belleville, Ont.: Mika 1977), 55–61; Nick Mika and Helma Mika, comp., *Belleville Centenary Flashback* (Belleville, Ont.: Mika 1978).

3 *The City of the Bay: Belleville and Her Industries*, Souvenir Industrial Number of *Daily Intelligencer*, 1909.

4 Interview with Drs Barbara and C.J. Wyatt at their home in Rome, Georgia, 11 February 1995, by author.

5 *The City of the Bay.*

6 I am greatly indebted to M.L. Barr and R.J. Rossiter for their excellent, detailed biographical essay on Collip. Barr and Rossiter, "James Bertram Collip, 1892–1965"; R.L. Noble, "Memories of James Bertram Collip," *Canadian Medical Association Journal* 93 (1965): 1357.

7 T.A. Reed, ed., *A History of the University of Trinity College, 1852–1952*, (Toronto: University of Toronto Press 1952); Barr and Rossiter, "James Bertram Collip," 236–8; "The Lit," *Trinity University Review* 24, no. 3: 57; David A. Keys, "James Bertram Collip," *Canadian Medical Association Journal* 93 (1965): 774–5; "The Science Club," *Trinity University Review* 26, no. 3: 56–7.

8 This portion is largely drawn from Sandra McRae's PhD thesis. Sandra McRae, "The 'Scientific Spirit' in Medicine at the University of Toronto, 1880–1910" (PhD thesis, University of Toronto, 1987); Abraham Flexner, *Medical Education in the United States and Canada: A Report to the Carnegie Foundation for the Advancement of Teaching* (New York: Carnegie Foundation for the Advancement of Teaching 1910), bulletin no. 4, 325–6.

9 Barr and Rossiter, "James Bertram Collip, 1892–1965," 237–8; interview with Drs Barbara and C.J. Wyatt, 11 February 1995, by author.

10 J.B. Collip, "Addison Lecture, Guys Hospital," 3.

11 Collip, "Addison Lecture, Guys Hospital," 3–7; J.B. Collip, "Some Observations on the Structure and Microchemistry of Nerve Cells" (MA thesis, University of Toronto, 1913); A.B. Macallum and J.B. Collop [sic],"A New Substance in Nerve Cells,"*Report of the British Association* 83 (1913): 673–4; *Trinity University Review* 26, no. 3 (December 1913): 61.

12 J.B. Collip, *On the Formation of Hydrochloric Acid in the Gastric Tubes of the Vertebrate Stomach*, University of Toronto Studies, Physiological Series, no. 35 (Toronto: University of Toronto Press 1920).

13 J.B. Collip, "Mind and the Cerebral Mechanism," *Trinity University Review* 26, no. 4 (January 1914): 79–81; McRae, "The 'Scientific Spirit' in Medicine," 132, 141.

14 "Trinity College Science Club," *Trinity University Review* 26, no. 4 (January 1914): 84; J.B. Collip, "Further Evidence of an Organic Evolution of Life," *Trinity University Review* 27, no. 4 (January 1915): 81–2; "The Theological Society," *Trinity University Review* 26, no. 5 (February 1914): 107.

15 Interview with Drs Barbara and C.J. Wyatt, 11 February 1995, by author. Photographs in the possession of the Wyatts.

16 Elise A. Corbet, *Frontiers of Medicine: A History of Medical Education and Research at the University of Alberta* (Edmonton, Alta: University of Alberta Press 1990), 15.

17 Corbet, *Frontiers of Medicine*, xiii–xx, 1–54, 168–73.

18 For examples of the experiences of a physician in the remote Peace River Region of Northern Alberta, see the story of Dr Mary Percy Jackson. Mary Percy Jackson, edited and with an introduction by Janice Dickin McGinnis, *Suitable for the Wilds: Letters from Northern Alberta, 1921–1931* (Toronto: University of Toronto Press 1995).

19 Interview of John Scott by Michael Bliss; John W. Scott, "Dr. J.B. Collip, Alberta period, 1915–1928," typescript, November 1965, Collip Correspondence, file "Library," Regional Collection, University of Western Ontario (hereafter UWO); Fred D. Locke and others to H.H. Moshier, 17 January 1916, 68–9–152, H.M. Tory Papers, University of Alberta Archives (hereafter UAA); J.B. Collip to H.M. Tory, 26 April 1916, 68–9–152, H.M. Tory Papers, UAA.

20 Corbet, *Frontiers of Medicine*, 15, 20; John W. Scott, "Dr. J.B. Collip, Alberta period"; Barr and Rossiter, "James Bertram Collip 1892–1965," 238; J.B. Collip, "Internal Secretions," *Canadian Medical Association Journal* 6 (1916): 1063–9.

21 Collip, "Addison Lecture, Guys Hospital," 3; Corbet, *Frontiers of Medicine*, 40–3.

22 J.B. Collip, Report of work, B.C. Biological Station, Departure Bay, 27 June–7 August 1916, Pacific Biological Station Archives, Nanaimo, B.C.; Barr and Rossiter, "James Bertram Collip, 1892–1965," 239; Collip, "Addison Lecture, Guys Hospital," 7–9.

23 Corbet, *Frontiers of Medicine*, 15, 20.

24 Barr and Rossiter, "James Bertram Collip, 1892–1965," 236; interview with Drs Barbara and C.J. Wyatt, 11 February 1995, by author.

25 Barr and Rossiter, "James Bertram Collip, 1892–1965," 239.

26 Collip, "Addison Lecture, Guys Hospital," 9–10; J.B. Collip, "Effect of Sleep upon the Alkali Reserve of the Plasma," *Journal of Biological*

Chemistry 41 (1920): 473–4; James Bertram Collip and P.L. Backus, "The Effect of Prolonged Hyperpnoea on the Carbon Dioxide Combining Power of the Plasma, the Carbon Dioxide Tension of Alveolar Air and the Excretion of Acid and Basic Phosphate and Ammonia by the Kidney," *American Journal of Physiology* 51 (1920): 568–79; idem, "The Alkali Reserve of the Blood Plasma, Spinal Fluid and Lymph," *American Journal of Physiology* 51 (1920): 551–67.

27 J.B. Collip, "Osmotic Pressure of Serum and Erythrocytes in Various Vertebrate Types as Determined by the Cryoscopic Method," *Journal of Biological Chemistry* 42 (1920): 207–12; idem, "Effect of Dilution on the Osmotic Pressure and the Electrical Conductivity of Whole Blood, Blood Serum, and Corpuscles," *Journal of Biological Chemistry* 42 (1920): 213–20; idem, "Osmotic Pressure of Tissue as Determined by the Cryoscopic Method," *Journal of Biological Chemistry* 42 (1920): 221–6; idem, "Maintenance of Osmotic Pressure within the Nucleus," *Journal of Biological Chemistry* 42 (1920): 227–36; idem, "Antagonism of Inhibitory Action of Adrenalin and Depression of Cardiac Vagus by a Constituent of Certain Tissue Extracts," *American Journal of Physiology* 53 (1920): 343–54; idem, "Reversal of Depressor Action of Small Doses of Adrenalin," *American Journal of Physiology* 55 (1921): 450–4; idem, "Antagonism of Depressor Action of Small Doses of Adrenalin by Tissue Extracts," *American Journal of Physiology* 53 (1920): 477–82.

28 Collip, "Addison Lecture, Guys Hospital," 7–9; idem, "The Alkali Reserve of Marine Fish and Invertebrates," *Journal of Biological Chemistry* 44 (1920): 329–44; idem, "Studies on Molluscan Celomic Fluid. Effect of change in environment on the carbon dioxide content of the celomic fluid. Anaerobic respiration in mya arenaria," *Journal of Biological Chemistry* 45 (1920): 23–49.

29 Whatever his research abilities may have been, it seems Downs was certainly an indifferent teacher. Corbet notes that he reportedly developed his lecture notes upon his arrival in 1920 and used them for the remainder of his teaching career. Corbet, *Frontiers of Medicine*, 14–5, 21–2, 35, 43; interview of John Scott by Michael Bliss; H.M. Tory to J.B. Collip, 29 August 1921, 68–9–144, H.M. Tory Papers, UAA.

30 Corbet suggests this. Corbet, *Frontiers of Medicine*, 43.

CHAPTER TWO

1 Hans Selye, *From Dream to Discovery: On Being a Scientist* (New York: McGraw-Hill 1964), 33.

2 J.B. Collip, DME Fellowship card, Rockefeller Archive Center.

3 Historian Marianne Gosztonyi Ainley discusses Tory's administration, utilitarian attitude towards science, and long-standing conflict with Collip's col-

league ornithologist William Rowan. Marianne Gosztonyi Ainley, *Restless Energy: A Biography of William Rowan, 1891–1957* (Montreal: Véhicule Press 1993), 121, 191.

4 H.M. Tory to J.B. Collip, 29 August 1921, 68–9–144, H.M. Tory Papers, UAA.

5 Michael Bliss, "J.B. Collip: A Forgotten Member of the Insulin Team," in *Essays in the History of Canadian Medicine*, ed. Wendy Mitchinson and Janice Dickin McGinnis (Toronto: McClelland and Stewart 1988), 110–25.

6 J.B. Collip to A.C. Rankin, 24 May 1921, 68–9–144, H.M. Tory Papers, UAA.

7 F.G. Banting notebook page, 31 October 1920, held by the Museum of the History of Health and Medicine, Toronto.

8 The story of Banting's pursuit of this idea is told in Michael Bliss's definitive and compelling account, *The Discovery of Insulin* (Toronto: McClelland and Stewart 1981); and much of my sketch of this episode depends on his study.

9 Bliss, *The Discovery of Insulin*, 25, 45–58.

10 Ibid., 57, 63–4.

11 Noble, "Memories of James Bertram Collip," 1356–64.

12 J.B. Collip, DME Fellowship card, Rockefeller Archive Center; Collip, "Addison Lecture, Guys Hospital," 11; idem, "A Further Study of the Respiratory Processes in Mya Arenaria and Other Marine Mollusca," *Journal of Biological Chemistry* 49 (1921): 297–310; J.B. Collip to H.M. Tory, 7 September 1921, 68–9–144, H.M. Tory Papers, UAA.

13 Ainley, *Restless Energy*, 191, referring to Trevor Levere's term "entrepreneurial scientific ideology." Trevor Levere, "What Is Canadian about Science in Canadian History?" in *Science, Technology and Canadian History*, ed. R.A. Jarrell and N.R. Ball (Waterloo, Ont.: Wilfrid Laurier University Press 1980), 20.

14 J.B. Collip to H.M. Tory, 19 June 1921, 68–9–144, H.M. Tory Papers, UAA.

15 H.M. Tory to J.B. Collip, 29 August 1921, 68–9–144, H.M. Tory Papers, UAA.

16 J.B. Collip to H.M. Tory, 19 October 1921, 68–9–144, H.M. Tory Papers, UAA.

17 H.M. Tory to J.B. Collip, 6 December 1921, 68–9–144, H.M. Tory Papers, UAA.

18 The description of the insulin work is largely drawn from the definitive account in Bliss, *Discovery of Insulin*, 85, 93.

19 Bliss, "Collip: A Forgotten Member of the Insulin Team," 114.

20 Bliss, *Discovery of Insulin*, 104–8.

21 J.B. Collip to H.M. Tory, 8 January 1922, 68–9–144, H.M. Tory Papers, UAA.

22 J.B. Collip to H.M. Tory, 8 January 1922, 68–9–144, H.M. Tory Papers, UAA.

23 H.M. Tory to J.B. Collip, 18 January 1922, 68–9–144, H.M. Tory Papers,
   UAA.

24 Bliss, *Discovery of Insulin*, 110–16.

25 Ibid., 108–13; O.H. Gaebler, "Letter to the Editor," *Bulletin of the Canadian Biochemical Society* 2, no. 3 (1965): 1.

26 Interview with Drs Barbara and C.J. Wyatt, 11 February 1995, by author;
   Margaret (Collip) McBride quoted in Marcia Mazur, "Insulin's Forgotten
   Man," *Diabetes Forecast*, May 1991: 48–9.

27 Bliss suggests that the breakthrough occurred after midnight on the 16th,
   based on a handwritten letter in the Collip papers listing Collip's contributions and apparently dating the isolation on 17 January. I've dated the event
   on 19 January because of a letter Collip wrote to Tory on 25 January in
   which he writes of a phenomenal break, saying "last Thursday Jan 19th I finally unearthed a method of isolating the internal secretion of the pancreas
   in a fairly pure and seemingly stable form suitable for human administration." J.B. Collip to H.M. Tory, 25 January 1922, 68–9–144, H.M. Tory
   Papers, UAA. Margaret (Collip) McBride is quoted in Marcia Mazur, "Insulin's Forgotten Man," as saying her father spoke years later about running
   in the halls in excitement and phoning his wife.

28 Bliss, *Discovery of Insulin*, 116–22.

29 Ibid., 11, 22–44.

30 J.B. Collip to H.M. Tory, 25 January 1922, 68–9–144, H.M. Tory Papers,
   UAA.

31 Bliss, *Discovery of Insulin*, 118–20.

32 Ibid., 129–40, 177–8.

33 Frederick Grant Banting, C.H. Best, J.B. Collip, and J.J.R. Macleod, "The
   Preparation of Pancreatic Extracts Containing Insulin," *Transactions of the
   Royal Society of Canada* 16, section 5 (1922): 27–9; Frederick Grant
   Banting, C.H. Best, J.B. Collip, J.J.R. Macleod, and E.C. Noble, "The Ef-
   fect of Insulin on Normal Rabbits and on Rabbits Rendered Hyperglycae-
   mic in Various Ways," *Transactions of the Royal Society of Canada* 16,
   section 5 (1922): 31–3; Frederick Grant Banting, C.H. Best, J.B. Collip,
   J. Hepburn, and J.J.R. Macleod, "The Effect Produced on the Respiratory
   Quotient by Injections of Insulin," *Transactions of the Royal Society of
   Canada* 16, section 5 (1922): 35–7; Frederick Grant Banting, C.H. Best,
   J.B. Collip, J.J.R. Macleod, and E.C. Noble, "The Effect of Insulin on the
   Percentage Amounts of Fat and Glycogen in the Liver and Other Organs of
   Diabetic Animals," *Transactions of the Royal Society of Canada* 16, section
   5 (1922): 39–42; Frederick Grant Banting, C.H. Best, J.B. Collip, and J.J.R.
   Macleod, "The Effect of Insulin on the Excretion of Ketone Bodies by the
   Diabetic Dog," *Transactions of the Royal Society of Canada* 16, section 5
   (1922): 43–4.

34 Bliss, "Collip: A Forgotten Member of the Insulin Team," 125; idem, "The Aetiology of the Discovery of Insulin," in *Health, Disease and Medicine: Essays in Canadian History*, ed. Charles G. Roland (Toronto: Hannah Institute for the History of Medicine 1984), 333–46.

CHAPTER THREE

1 A.M. Hanson to H. Cushing, 15 April 1925, box 2, file "Cushing," A.M. Hanson Papers, Owen Wangesteen Historical Library of Biology and Medicine, University of Minnesota (hereafter Hanson Papers).

2 Bliss, *Discovery of Insulin*, 147, 219; idem, "J.B. Collip, a Forgotten Member of the Insulin Team," 121–5; Corbet, *Frontiers of Medicine*, 45–6.

3 Bliss, *Discovery of Insulin*, 219, 229–32.

4 The royalties were divided among the University of Toronto, Collip, Banting, and Best, for the purpose of medical research. By 1927 the insulin royalties paid to Collip amounted to $13,648. Agreement between the Governors of the University of Toronto and James Bertram Collip, 1 July 1923, J.B. Collip Papers, Regional Collection, UWO; J.B. Collip to C.F. Martin, 9 December 1927, RG 2, container 136, file 3974, Principal's Papers, McGill University Archives (hereafter MUA); Corbet, *Frontiers of Medicine*, 45.

5 Corbet, *Frontiers of Medicine*, xiii–xx, 1–54, 168–73; N.P. Colwell to Henry Marshall Tory, 16 November 1922, RG 3, file 68-9-148, H.M. Tory Papers UAA. J.B. Collip to H.M. Tory, 10 July [1926], and H.M. Tory to J.B. Collip, 16 July 1926, both in 68–9–144, H.M. Tory Papers, UAA.

6 J.B. Collip to H.M. Tory, 21 April 1922, 68–9–144, H.M. Tory Papers, UAA; Bliss, *Discovery of Insulin*, 156.

7 H.M. Tory to R.M. Pearce, 28 June 1923, Rockefeller Foundation (hereafter RF) RG 1.1, 427A, box 8, folder 66, Rockefeller Archive Center (hereafter RAC).

8 Corbet, *Frontiers of Medicine*, 34–5, 170–2.

9 A.B. Macallum to A.G. Huntsman, 16 January 1925, B78–0010, box 27, file 4, A.G. Huntsman Papers, University of Toronto Archives (hereafter UTA).

10 Sir Arthur Currie to J.B. Collip, 16 April 1924, RG 2, container 67, file 1258, Principal's Papers, MUA.

11 J.B. Collip to Sir Arthur Currie, 25 April [1924], RG 2, container 67, file 1258, Principal's Papers, MUA.

12 Corbet, *Frontiers of Medicine*, 46.

13 Bliss, *Discovery of Insulin*, 181–7.

14 J.B. Collip, "The Occurrence of Ketone Bodies in the Urine of Normal Rabbits in a Condition of Hypoglycemia Following the Administration of

Insulin – A Condition of Acute Acidosis Experimentally Produced," *Journal of Biological Chemistry* 55 (1923): xxxviii–xxxix; idem, "The Original Method as Used for the Isolation of Insulin in Semipure Form for the Treatment of the First Clinical Cases," *Journal of Biological Chemistry* 55 (1923): xl–xli; idem, "Delayed Manifestation of the Physiological Effects of Insulin Following the Administration of Certain Pancreatic Extracts," *American Journal of Physiology* 63 (1923): 391–2; idem, "The Demonstration of an Insulin-like Substance in the Tissues of the Clam (Mya Arenaria)," *Journal of Biological Chemistry* 55 (1923): xxxix.

15 J.B. Collip, "The Demonstration of a Hormone in Plant Tissues to Be Known as 'Glucokinin,'" *Proceedings of the Society for Experimental Biology and Medicine* 20 (1923): 321–3.

16 J.B. Collip, "Effect of Plant Extracts on Blood Sugar," *Nature* 111 (1923): 571.

17 Bliss, *Discovery of Insulin*, 185.

18 J.B. Collip, "Glucokinin. A New Hormone Present in Plant Tissue. Preliminary Paper," *Journal of Biological Chemistry* 56 (1923): 513–43.

19 J.B. Collip, "Glucokinin. Second Paper," *Journal of Biological Chemistry* 57 (1923): 65–78.

20 J.B. Collip, "Glucokinin. An Apparent Synthesis in the Normal Animal of a Hypoglycemia-producing Principle. Animal passage of the principle," *Journal of Biological Chemistry* 58 (1923): 163–208.

21 J.B. Collip, "Animal Passage Hypoglycaemia," *Proceedings of the Society for Experimental Biology and Medicine* 24 (1927): 731–2.

22 J.B. Collip, "The Effect of Insulin on the Oxygen Consumption of Certain Marine Fish and Invertebrates," *American Journal of Physiology* 72 (1925): 181–2.

23 The term "isolation" is used by some contemporaries and later commentators. In fact, a more accurate description of Collip's accomplishment is the preparation of an active extract of the hormone. The parathyroid hormone was not isolated in pure form until the 1950s, when it was discovered that the extracts prepared according to Hanson's and Collip's method contained biologically active but unstable fragments of the hormone. Paul L. Munson, "Parathyroid Hormone and Calcitonin," in *Endocrinology: People and Ideas*, ed. S.M. McCann (Bethesda, Md.: American Physiological Society 1988), 265–8; Howard Rasmussen and Lyman C. Craig, "The Parathyroid Polypeptides," *Recent Progress in Hormone Research* 18 (1962): 269–95; Howard Rasmussen, "Chemistry of Parathyroid Hormone," in *The Parathyroids: Proceedings of a Symposium on Advances in Parathyroid Research*, ed. Roy O. Greep and Roy V. Talmage (Springfield, Ill.: Charles C. Thomas 1961), 60–9; G.D. Aurbach, "Purification of Parathyroid Hormone," in *The Parathyroids: Proceedings of a Symposium on Advances in*

Parathyroid Research, ed. Roy O. Greep and Roy V. Talmage (Springfield, Ill.: Charles C. Thomas 1961), 51–9.

24 A description of their work first appeared in Alison Li, "J.B. Collip, A.M. Hanson, and the Isolation of the Parathyroid Hormone, or Endocrines and Enterprise," *Journal of the History of Medicine and Allied Sciences* 47, no. 2 (1992): 405–38.

25 Merriley Borell, "Organotherapy, British Physiology, and Discovery of the Internal Secretions," *Journal of the History of Biology* 9 (1976): 235–68; idem, "Brown-Séquard's Organotherapy and Its Appearance in America at the End of the Nineteenth Century," *Bulletin of the History of Medicine* 50 (1976): 309–20; idem, "Setting the Standards for a New Science: Edward Schäfer and Endocrinology," *Medical History* 22 (1978): 282–90.

26 Diana Long Hall, "The Critic and the Advocate: Contrasting British Views on the State of Endocrinology in the Early 1920's," *Journal of the History of Biology* 9 (1976): 269–85.

27 Victor Cornelius Medvei, *A History of Endocrinology* (Lancaster, England: MTP Press 1982), 501–7; Hans Lisser, "The Endocrine Society: First Forty Years (1917–1957)," *Endocrinology* 80 (1967): 5–28.

28 Jonathan Liebenau, *Medical Science and Medical Industry: The Formation of the American Pharmaceutical Industry* (Baltimore, Md.: Johns Hopkins University Press 1987), 30–47.

29 John P. Swann, *Academic Scientists and the Pharmaceutical Industry: Co-operative Research in Twentieth-Century America* (Baltimore, Md.: Johns Hopkins University Press 1987), 118–49; Bliss, *Discovery of Insulin*, 137–41, 240–1.

30 The University of Minnesota held the patent for thyroxine, isolated by Edward Kendall in 1915; the University of Wisconsin held the patent for the method of producing vitamin D by irradiation developed by Harry Steenbock. Liebenau, *Medical Science and Medical Industry*, 1–10, 96, 125–34; Richard H. Shryock, *American Medical Research* (New York: Commonwealth Fund 1947), 140–4; Bliss, *Discovery of Insulin*, 139–40, 174–81; Rima D. Apple, "Patenting University Research: Harry Steenbock and the Wisconsin Alumni Research Foundation," *Isis* 80 (1989): 375–94; Charles Weiner, "Patenting and Academic Research: Historical Case Studies," in *Owning Scientific and Technical Information: Value and Ethical Issues*, ed. Vivian Weil and John W. Snapper (New Brunswick, N.J.: Rutgers University Press 1989), 87–109.

31 William S. McCann, "Parathyroid Therapy," *Journal of the American Medical Association* 83 (1924): 1847.

32 William G. MacCallum and Carl Voegtlin, "On the Relation of Tetany to the Parathyroid Glands and to Calcium Metabolism," *Journal of Experimental Medicine* 11 (1909): 118–51.

33 D. Noël Paton and Leonard Findlay, "The Parathyroids: Tetania Parathyreopriva: Its Nature, Cause and Relation to Idiopathic Tetany," parts 1–4,
Quarterly Journal of Experimental Physiology 10 (1916): 203–31, 233–42,
243–314, 315–344; Eran Dolev, "A Gland in Search of a Function: The
Parathyroid Glands and the Explanations of Tetany 1903–1926," *Journal
of the History of Medicine and Allied Sciences* 42 (1987): 186–98.

34 John W. Scott, "Biographical Sketch, Dr. J.B. Collip, Alberta Period," 3–4;
J.B. Collip, "The Significance of the Calcium-Ion in the Cell – Experimental
Tetany," *Canadian Medical Association Journal* 10 (1920): 935–7; J.B. Col-
lip and P.L. Backus, "The Effect of Prolonged Hyperpnoea on the Carbon
Dioxide Combining Power of the Plasma, the Carbon Dioxide Tension of
Alveolar Air and the Excretion of Acid and Basic Phosphate and Ammonia
by the Kidney," *American Journal of Physiology* 51 (1920): 568–79; L.B.
Winter and W. Smith, "On a Possible Relation between the Pancreas and
the Parathyroids," *Journal of Physiology* 58 (1923–24): 108–10.

35 J.B. Collip, "The Extraction of a Parathyroid Hormone Which Will Prevent
or Control Parathyroid Tetany and Which Regulates the Level of Blood
Calcium," *Journal of Biological Chemistry* 63 (1925): 395–438.

36 D.L. Thomson, "Dr James Bertram Collip," *Canadian Journal of Biochem-
istry and Physiology* 35, suppl. (1957): 3–7; Noble, "Memories of James
Bertram Collip," 1359; interview of Robert Noble, 5 June 1990, by author,
Vancouver, B.C.

37 Collip, "The Extraction of a Parathyroid Hormone Which Will Prevent or
Control Parathyroid Tetany," 433.

38 J.B. Collip, E.P. Clark, and J.W. Scott, "The Effect of a Parathyroid Hormone on Normal Animals," *Journal of Biological Chemistry* 63 (1925):
439–60. Collip and Clark modified the existing Kramer-Tisdall method of
serum calcium determination so that it provided results consistent within
plus or minus 0.2 mg per 100 cc. E.P. Clark and J.B. Collip, "A Study of the
Tisdall Method for the Determination of Blood Serum Calcium with a Suggested Modification," *Journal of Biological Chemistry* 63 (1925): 461–4;
J.B. Collip, "Addison Lecture, Guys Hospital," 10–11.

39 J.B. Collip and D.B. Leitch, "A Case of Tetany Treated with Parathyrin,"
Canadian Medical Association Journal 15 (1925): 59–60; J.B. Collip,
"Clinical Use of the Parathyroid Hormone," *Canadian Medical Association
Journal* 15 (1925): 1158.

40 G.H.A. Clowes to H.M. Tory, 24 April 1925, RG 3, file 68-9-144, H.M.
Tory Papers, UAA.

41 Collip, "The Extraction of a Parathyroid Hormone Which Will Prevent or
Control Tetany," 437.

42 Adolph Martin Hanson, "A Brief History of the Family of Adolph
Melanchton Hanson and Marie Lucile Boxrud as Recorded by Their Son,"
unpublished manuscript, Hanson Papers.

43 He may also have gained some familiarity with goitre surgery as a result of his friendly association with William and Charles Mayo of the Mayo Clinic in nearby Rochester, where many such procedures were carried out. A.M. Hanson to E.O. Ellingson, 4 September 1922, box 3, file "Parathyroid 1922," Hanson Papers.

44 He changed the method for one of the standard tests, using hydrochloric acid instead of sulphuric acid just for the sake of experiment. A.M. Hanson to E.O. Ellingson, 22 January 1923, box 3, file "Parathyroid 1923," Hanson papers; A.M. Hanson to E.O. Ellingson, 12 February 1923, box 3, file "Parathyroid 1923," Hanson Papers; Adolph M. Hanson, "An Elementary Chemical Study of the Parathyroid Glands of Cattle," *Military Surgeon* 53 (March 1923): 280–4; Adolph M. Hanson, "Notes on the Hydrochloric X of the Bovine Parathyroid," *Military Surgeon* 53 (April 1923): 434.

45 A.M. Hanson to E.O. Ellingson, 2 February 1923, file "Parathyroid 1923"; typed laboratory notes beginning "Goiter case – October 4, 1922"; A.B. Bell to A.M. Hanson, 22 August 1923; and A.M. Hanson to E.O. Ellingson, 30 November 1923, all in box 3, file "Parathyroid 1923" Hanson Papers.

46 E.O. Ellingson, A.W. Bell, and Adolph M. Hanson, "Experiments with an Active Extract of Parathyroid," *Proceedings of the Society for Experimental Biology and Medicine* 21 (1923–24): 274–5; Adolph M. Hanson, "The Hydrochloric X of the Bovine Parathyroid and Its Phosphotungstic Acid Precipitate," *Military Surgeon* 54 (February 1924): 218–19; Adolph M. Hanson, "Parathyroid Preparations," *Military Surgeon* 54 (May 1924): 554–60; Adolph M. Hanson, "Parathyroid Active Preparations of Parathyroid Other Than That of the Desiccated Gland," *Military Surgeon* 54 (December 1924): 701–18.

47 A.M. Hanson to E.O. Ellingson, 22 January 1923; E.O. Ellingson to A.M. Hanson, 19 July 1924; A.M. Hanson to E.O. Ellingson, 4 September 1924; and A.M. Hanson to E.O. Ellingson, 15 November 1924, all in box 3, file "Parathyroid 1924," Hanson Papers.

48 J.B. Collip and E.P. Clark, "Further Studies on the Physiological Action of a Parathyroid Hormone," *Journal of Biological Chemistry* 64 (1925): 485–507; idem, "Further Studies on the Parathyroid Hormone: Second Paper," *Journal of Biological Chemistry* 66 (1925): 133–7; idem, "Concerning the Relation of Guanidine to Parathyroid Tetany," *Journal of Biological Chemistry* 67 (1926): 679–87.

49 J.B. Collip, "The Therapeutic Value of the Parathyroid Hormone," *Journal of the American Medical Association* 87 (18 September 1926): 908–10; Collip and Clark, "Further Studies on the Parathyroid Hormone: Second Paper," 134.

50 William S. McCann, "Parathyroid Therapy," *Journal of the American Medical Association* 88 (19 February 1927): 566.

51 Ibid., 566–7; J.B. Collip, "The Calcium Mobilizing Hormone of the Parathyroid Glands: Chemistry and Physiology, *Journal of the American Medical Association* 88 (19 February 1927): 565–6.

52 According to Collip's initial publication, the preparation of the extract entailed (1) boiling the glands in 5 percent hydrochloric acid for one hour, (2) performing two isoelectric precipitations to pull out other proteins, and (3) filtering or centrifuging to remove the precipitates. Hanson's method consisted of boiling the glands in 10 parts per 1,000 hydrochloric acid for two hours and filtering the result. Collip's HCl concentration is approximately 1.4 N or about 14 times Hanson's. Later studies seem to have shown that the best extraction occurs at about 0.2 N.

53 A.M. Hanson to H. Cushing, 15 April 1925, box 2, file "Cushing"; and A.M. Hanson to A.M. Hjort, 5 October 1925, box 3, file "Parathyroid 1925," both in Hanson Papers.

54 A.M. Hanson to E.O. Ellingson, 27 January 1924 [should be dated 1925], box 3, file "Parathyroid 1924," Hanson Papers; A.M. Hanson, "The Hormone of the Parathyroid Gland," *Proceedings of the Society for Experimental Biology and Medicine* 22 (1925): 560–1; idem, "The Hormone of the Parathyroid Gland – Changes in the Blood Serum Calcium of Thyroparathyroidectomized Dogs Modified by the Bovine Hydrochloric X," *Minnesota Medicine* 8 (May 1925): 283–5; A.M. Hjort, S.C. Robinson, and F.H. Tendick, "An Extract Obtained from the External Bovine Parathyroid Glands Capable of Inducing Hypercalcemia in Normal and Thyreoparathyroprivic Dogs," *Journal of Biological Chemistry* 65 (1925): 117–28. A.M. Hjort to A.M. Hanson, 10 April 1925, and A.M. Hjort to A.M. Hanson, 11 July 1925, both in box 3, file "Parathyroid 1925," Hanson Papers.

55 Bliss, *Discovery of Insulin*; idem, *Banting, A Biography* (Toronto: McClelland and Stewart 1984).

56 J.B. Collip, "The Internal Secretion of the Parathyroid Glands," *Proceedings of the National Academy of Science* 11 (1925): 484–5; Collip and Clark, "Further Studies on the Physiological Action of a Parathyroid Hormone," 506.

57 G.H.A. Clowes to J.B. Collip, telegram, 21 April 1925, and G.H.A. Clowes to J.B. Collip, telegram, 22 April 1925, both in RG 3, file 68-9-144, H.M. Tory Papers, UAA.

58 G.H.A. Clowes to H.M. Tory, 24 April 1925, RG 3, file 68-9-144, H.M. Tory Papers, UAA.

59 A.M. Hanson to H. Cushing, 15 April 1925, box 2, file "Cushing," Hanson Papers. H.W. Rhodehamel to A.M. Hanson, 14 May 1925; H.W. Rhodehamel to A.M. Hanson, 14 May 1925; and A.J. Hjort to A.M. Hanson, 28 April 1925, all in box 3, file "Parathyroid 1925," Hanson Papers.

60 H.M. Tory to W.A. Puckner, 5 October 1925, RG 3, file 68-9-144, H.M. Tory Papers, UAA.

61 A.M. Hjort to A.M. Hanson, 8 April 1925, 10 April 1925, 15 April 1925, and 24 April 1925, box 3, file "Parathyroid 1925," Hanson Papers.

62 A.M. Hanson to H.J. Shaughnessy, 21 November 1925, box 3, file "Parathyroid 1925," Hanson Papers. A.J. Hjort to A.M. Hanson, 6 May 1926, and A.M. Hanson to H.J. Hjort, 22 May 1926, both in box 3, file "Parathyroid 1926," Hanson Papers. A.M. Hanson to L.G. Rowntree, 17 October 1934, box 1, file "Thymus 1934"; A.M. Hanson to L.K. Kast, 26 November 1935, box 1, file "Thymus 1935"; and case notes beginning 8-1-27, box 3, file "Parathyroid 1927," all in Hanson Papers.

63 The unit used in the U.S. Pharmacopoeia XVI revision was similar in size to Hanson's but used the rise in serum calcium in normal dogs. For an example of one unfortunate researcher whose work was complicated by having to use both the Collip extract measured in the Collip unit and the Hanson extract measured in the Hanson unit, see Robert Burrows, "Variations Produced in Bones of Growing Rats by Parathyroid Extracts," *American Journal of Anatomy* 62 (1938): 237–90. Collip and Clark, "Further Studies on the Physiological Action of a Parathyroid Hormone"; Adolph M. Hanson, "The Standardization of Parathyroid Activity," *Journal of the American Medical Association* 90 (10 March 1928): 747–8; J.B. Collip, "The Internal Secretion of the Parathyroid Glands," *International Clinics* 3 (1925): 77–80; copy of patent Interference No. 56,067 Final Hearing, 5 March 1931, box 3, file "Parathyroid 1931," Hanson Papers; Louis Berman, "A Crystalline Substance from the Parathyroid Glands That Influences the Calcium Content of the Blood," *Proceedings of the Society for Experimental Biology and Medicine* 21 (1923–24): 465; idem, "Separation of an Internal Secretion of the Parathyroid Glands," *Laboratory and Clinical Medicine* 11 (1925–26): 11, 412–13; idem, "The Effect of a Protein-Free Acid-Alcohol Extract of the Parathyroid Glands upon the Calcium Content of the Blood and the Electrical Irritability of the Nerves of Parathyroidectomized and Normal Animals," *American Journal of Physiology* 57 (1925–26): 358–65. In contrast to Hanson, Berman did not argue that he had developed the method of extraction earlier than Collip. Rather, he challenged Collip's claim to originality in conceiving and executing the idea of obtaining the internal secretion of the parathyroid. Louis Berman, "Priority in the Isolation of Parathyroid Hormone," *Journal of the American Medical Association* 89 (1927): 310–11.

64 Hanson's accusation against Collip appears in a manuscript prepared but not accepted for publication. A.M. Hanson, "The Parathyroid: Retrospect and Prospect," unpublished manuscript, 27 June 1927, box 3, file "Parathyroid 1927," Hanson Papers. Hanson submitted papers to the *Journal of the American Medical Association* and the *New York Medical Journal* in the fall of 1923, but they were not accepted. A.M. Hanson to E.O. Ellingson, 5 November 1923, and A.M Hanson to E.O. Ellingson, 30 November

1923, both in box 3, file "Parathyroid 1923," Hanson Papers. I am indebted to an anonymous reviewer of the *Journal of the History of Medicine and Allied Sciences* who brought this to my attention. His detailed comments and thorough analysis helped me sharpen my discussion of this question.

65 G.H.A. Clowes to H.M. Tory, 24 April 1925, RG 3, file 68-9-144, H.M. Tory Papers, UAA.

66 Collip, "The Extraction of a Parathyroid Hormone Which Will Prevent or Control Parathyroid Tetany," 437.

67 D.K. O'Donovan, "Some Reminiscences of Canadian Endocrinology," *Journal of the Irish Medical Association* 69 (26 June 1976): 298.

68 A.M. Hanson to L.G. Rowntree, 24 March 1925, box 1, file "Thymus 1933," Hanson Papers.

69 Lisser, "The Endocrine Society," 5–6.

70 Harvey Cushing, "Disorders of the Pituitary Gland: Retrospective and Prospective," *Journal of the American Medical Association* 76 (18 June 1921): 1721–6.

71 Editorial, "Parathyrin (Collip)," *Endocrinology* 9 (1925): 242.

72 "What's a Monkey Gland? It's Largely Buncombe," *Star Weekly* (Toronto), 6 June 1925. Barbara Clow argues that the Canadian medical community of this period was far slower to take a stand against irregular practitioners and quacks, whether out of tolerance or apathy. Canadian practitioners did not attempt to rally public support against "irregulars," relying on government legislation to restrict their activities. Barbara Clow, "Mahlon William Locke: 'Toe-twister,'" *Canadian Bulletin of Medical History* 9 (1992): 17–39.

73 F.C. McLean, keynote address, and G.D. Aurbach, "Purification of Parathyroid Hormone," both in Greep and Talmage, eds, *The Parathyroids*, 17, 51.

74 Morrell may have been a claimant for Swan-Meyer Company. A representative of the firm visited Hanson on 7 September 1925, indicating that he might face a patent interference from them because they had a product called "Parathyrin" on the market. A.M. Hanson to A.J. Hjort, 7 September 1925, box 3, file "Parathyroid 1925"; and Preliminary Statement on Patent Interference No. 56068, 19 December 1927, box 3, "Parathyroid 1927," both in Hanson Papers.

75 Copy of Patent Interference No. 56,067, Final Hearing, 5 March 1931, box 3, file "Parathyroid 1931," Hanson Papers.

76 A.M. Hanson to A.J. Andresen, 22 October 1928, box 3, "Parathyroid 1928"; and C.B. Zewadski to A.M. Hanson, 14 November 1932, box 3, file "Parathyroid 1932," both in Hanson Papers.

77 A.M. Hanson to L.G. Rowntree, 20 June 1933, box 1, file "Thymus 1933," Hanson Papers.

78 Adolph M. Hanson, "Physiology of the Parathyroid," *Journal of the American Medical Association* 105 (13 July 1935): 113–14; A.M. Hanson to L.G. Rowntree, 8 February 1933, 13 February 1933, and 16 February 1933, all in box 1, file "Thymus 1933," Hanson Papers; Nate Cardarelli, "Dr. Adolph Hanson and Karkinolysin," unpublished manuscript, January 1986; Nate F. Cardarelli and Bernadette M. Cardarelli, "Thymic Extract (Hanson): An Old Controversy Revisited," unpublished manuscript. Professor Cardarelli, of the Engineering and Science Technology Division, University of Akron, kindly allowed me to read the two manuscripts dealing with Hanson's later work on the thymus gland.

79 R.V. Talmage to J.B. Collip, 8 September 1959, Collip Correspondence, file 3, Regional Collection, UWO. Collip's later research on the physiology of the parathyroid hormone, particularly his disagreement with endocrinologist Fuller Albright, is discussed in Theodore B. Schwartz, "Giants with Tunnel Vision: The Albright-Collip Controversy," *Perspectives in Biology and Medicine* 34 (1991): 327–46; and Christiane Sinding, "Clinical Research and Basic Science: The Development of the Concept of End-Organ Resistance to a Hormone," *Journal of the History of Medicine and Allied Sciences* 45 (1990): 198–232.

80 Munson, "Parathyroid Hormone and Calcitonin," 252.

81 A.M. Hanson to L.G. Rowntree, 21 April 1933, box 1, file "Thymus 1933," Hanson Papers; D.L. Thomson and J.B. Collip, "The Hormone of the Parathyroid Glands," *International Clinics* 4 (1933): 102–13.

CHAPTER FOUR

1 J.B. Collip to C.F. Martin, 9 December [1927], RG 2, container 136, file 3874, Principal's Papers, MUA.

2 Sir Arthur Currie to J.B. Collip, 16 April 1924, and J.B. Collip to Sir Arthur W. Currie, 25 April [1924], both in RG 2, container 67, file 1258, Principal's Papers, MUA.

3 C.F. Martin to J.B. Collip, 9 August 1927, and L.G. Rowntree to J.B. Collip, 11 August 1927, both in J.B. Collip Papers, MS Collection 269, item 2, Fisher Rare Book Library, UT. Jack Collip, in an interview by Michael Bliss with Collip's daughter Barbara, John Scott, Mrs Scott, Rube Sandin, Bruce Collier, and Professor Shaner, notes, Edmonton, 4 October 1980; interview with Harold Ettinger, c. 1970, by Robert Noble, tape recording.

4 J.B. Collip to H.M. Tory, 30 August 1927, H.M Tory Papers, RG 3, file 68-9-144, UAA; J.B. Collip to C.F. Martin, 9 December [1927], RG 2, container 136, file 3874, Principal's Papers, MUA; Sir Arthur Currie to J.B. Collip, 27 September 1927, J.B. Collip Papers, MS Collection 269, item 2, Fisher Rare Book Library, UT.

5 I.M Rabinowitch to O.F. Denstedt, 10 March 1969, in MG 1031, AC 2049, O.F. Denstedt Papers, MUA. C.F. Martin to J.B. Collip, 20 October 1927, and J.B. Collip to Sir Arthur Currie, 8 November 1927, both in J.B. Collip Papers, MS Collection 269, item 2, Fisher Rare Book Library, UT.

6 J.B. Collip to Sir Arthur Currie, 8 November 1927, RG 2, container 67, file 1258, Principal's Papers, MUA; J.B. Collip to C.F. Martin, 9 December [1927], RG 2, container 136, file 3874, Principal's Papers, MUA.

7 Collip wrote in 1947, "I would like to state most emphatically how much I personally owe to him, and in like manner, my Department, and the University, for the part he played during the early years of my McGill tenure when we developed new and useful therapeutic agents for which, on the financial side, there has been a handsome reward in the establishment and growth of several special research funds under my control." J.B. Collip to Wm Bentley, 31 January 1947, MS Collection 269, item 4, Collip Papers, Fisher Rare Book Library, UT.

8 McRae, "The 'Scientific Spirit,' " 251–97.

9 Marianne Pauline Fedunkiw Stevens, "Dollars and Change: The Effect of Rockefeller Foundation Funding on Canadian Medical Education at the University of Toronto, McGill University, and Dalhousie University" (PhD thesis, University of Toronto, 2000), 153–93.

10 H.E. MacDermont, "The Rockefeller Benefactions," RG 2, container 68, file 1298, Principal's Papers, MUA.

11 Harvey Cushing, quoted by O.F. Denstedt. O.F. Denstedt, "The Evolution of Biochemistry at McGill," typescript, MG 1031, O.F. Denstedt Papers, MUA.

12 Wilder Penfield, "Dr. Penfield Describes How His Work at McGill Began," 147–8; and D. Sclater Lewis, "McGill's First Full-time Dean of Medicine: Dr. 'Charlie' Martin," 136–8, both in *The McGill You Knew: An Anthology of Memories, 1920–1960*, ed. Edgar Andrew Collard (Toronto: Longman Canada 1975).

13 Dorothy McMurry, *Four Principals of McGill: A Memoir, 1929–1963* (Montreal: Graduates' Society of McGill University 1974), 17–18; Daniel G. Dancocks, *Sir Arthur Currie: A Biography* (Toronto: Methuen 1985), 212–85; Hugh M. Urquhart, *Arthur Currie: The Biography of a Great Canadian* (Toronto: J.M. Dent & Sons 1950), 306.

14 C.F. Martin to Sir Arthur Currie, 25 October 1928, 7 February 1929, and 7 December 1929, all in RG 2, container 56, file 831, Principal's Papers, MUA (emphasis in the original).

15 Edward H. Bensley, *McGill Medical Luminaries* (Montreal: Osler Library 1990), 163–4; J.B. Collip to the Secretary of the Court, 13 February 1935, D.L. Thomson Papers, MG 2050, Acc 2049-778, MUA.

16 J.B. Collip, to C.F. Martin, 26 July [1930], RG 38, container 6, file 133, Faculty of Medicine records, MUA. J.B. Collip, "A Non-specific Pressor

Substance," *Transactions of the Royal Society of Canada* 22 (1928): 181–4; idem, "A Non-specific Pressor Substance," *American Journal of Physiology* 85 (1928): 360–1; idem, "A Non-Specific Pressor Principle Derived from a Variety of Tissues," *Journal of Physiology* 66 (1928): 416–30.

17 Bertold P. Wiesner and Norah M. Sheard, *Maternal Behaviour in the Rat* (Edinburgh: Oliver and Boyd 1933), vii–ix; J.B. Collip, "The Ovary-Stimulating Hormone of the Placenta: Preliminary Paper," *Canadian Medical Association Journal* 22 (1930): 216; idem, "The Ovary Stimulating Hormone of the Placenta," *Nature* 125 (1930): 444.

18 This hormone was later termed "chorionic gonadotrophin" because it was produced in the chorionic villi of the placenta. Victor Cornelius Medvei, *A History of Endocrinology* (Lancaster: MTP Press 1982), 406–9; A.S. Parkes, "The Rise of Reproductive Endocrinology, 1926–1940," in *Sex, Science and Society* (Newcastle-upon-Tyne: Oriel Press 1966), 30–1.

19 Medvei, *A History of Endocrinology*, 396–401.

20 Merriley Borell, "Organotherapy and the Emergence of Reproductive Endocrinology," *Journal of the History of Biology* 18 (1985): 11–12, 14.

21 J.B. Collip, "Further Observations on an Ovary-Stimulating Hormone of the Placenta," *Canadian Medical Association Journal* 22 (1930): 761–74.

22 Collip, "The Ovary-Stimulating Hormone of the Placenta: Preliminary Paper"; J.B. Collip to W.J. McKenna, 22 November 1938, Collip Papers, MS 269, item 3, Fisher Rare Book Library, UT.

23 J.B. Collip, "The Ovary Stimulating Hormone of the Placenta," *Nature* 125 (1930): 444; A.D. Campbell and J.B. Collip, "On the Clinical Use of the Ovary-Stimulating Hormone of the Placenta: Preliminary Report," *Canadian Medical Association Journal* 22 (1930): 219–20.

24 Neville Terry, *The Royal Vic: The Story of Montreal's Royal Victoria Hospital 1894–1994* (Montreal & Kingston: McGill-Queen's University Press 1994), 116–19.

25 Bensley *McGill Medical Luminaries*, 71–2; Nelly Oudshoorn, "On the Making of Sex Hormones: Research Materials and the Production of Knowledge," *Social Studies of Science* 20 (1990): 5–33.

26 "Important Discovery at McGill University," 12 February 1930, RG 2, container 67, file 1259, Principal's Papers; and C.F. Martin to Frank L. Horsfall, 19 February 1930, RG 38, container 6, file 133, Faculty of Medicine records, both in MUA.

27 Fuller Albright to J.B. Collip, 6 March 1930, Fuller Albright Papers, box 11, file " 'C' Inactive Correspondence," Francis A. Countway Library, Harvard Medical School; George H. Brooke to C.F. Martin, 11 March 1930, RG 38, container 6, file 133, Faculty of Medicine records, MUA.

28 J.B. Collip to H.H. Dale, 27 March 1930, RG 38, container 6, file 133, Faculty of Medicine records, MUA.

29 Collip, "Further Observations on an Ovary-Stimulating Hormone of the Placenta," 761; J.B. Collip to C.F. Martin, 25 April [1930], RG 38, container 6, file 133, Faculty of Medicine records, MUA.

30 Josiah K. Lilly to Sir Arthur Currie, 1 February 1930; Sir Arthur Currie to Josiah K. Lilly, 5 February 1930; Sir Arthur Currie, memo, 15 March 1930; W.A.S. Ayerst to J.B. Collip, 10 February 1930; and Sir Arthur Currie to Ayerst, McKenna & Harrison, 12 February 1930, all in RG 2, container 67, file 1259, Principal's Papers, MUA. J.C. Simpson to F. Cyril James, 13 December 1940, RG 38, container 6, file 133, Faculty of Medicine records, MUA. As the Eli Lilly & Company archives are now closed to outside researchers, it is difficult to ascertain the reasons Lilly did not pursue this project.

31 *Thirty-Five Years in the Pharmaceutical Manufacturing Industry in Canada* (Montreal: Ayerst, McKenna & Harrison Ltd 1961), 3–4.

32 *Thirty-Five Years*, 14; J.C. Simpson to F. Cyril James, 13 December 1940, RG 38, container 6, file 133, Faculty of Medicine records, MUA; Magnus Pyke, *The Six Lives of Pyke* (Toronto: J.M. Dent & Sons 1981), 62–3.

33 *Standard Dictionary of Canadian Biography*, vol. 2: *1875–1937*, 249–51.

34 Joseph Schull, *The Century of the Sun* (Toronto: Macmillan 1971); Michael Bliss, *Northern Enterprise* (Toronto: McClelland and Stewart 1987), 270–7.

35 *Canadian Who's Who, 1936–37* (Toronto: Times Publishing Co. 1937), 656; Schull, *The Century of the Sun*, 65; "T.B. Macaulay," obituary, *Globe and Mail* (Toronto), 4 April 1942. Macaulay's endowment provided an income of £2,100 per annum; Macaulay also donated £5,000 for the purchase of a farm. *Edinburgh University Calendar*, 1931–32, 701.

36 Sir Arthur Currie to C.F. Martin, 23 April 1930, RG 2, container 66, file 1229, Principal's Papers, MUA.

37 Sir Arthur Currie to C.F. Martin, 23 April 1930, RG 2, container 66, file 1229, Principal's Papers, MUA.

38 Sir Arthur Currie to C.F. Martin, 12 May 1930, RG 38, container 6, file 133, Faculty of Medicine records, MUA.

39 Sir Arthur Currie to C.F. Martin, 12 May 1930, RG 38, container 6, file 133, Faculty of Medicine records, MUA; *Edinburgh University Calendar*, 1933–34, 22; ibid., 1932–33, 383; ibid., 1931–32, 704.

40 J.B. Collip to C.F. Martin, 25 April [1930], RG 38, container 6, file 133, Faculty of Medicine records, MUA; Collip, "The Ovary-Stimulating Hormone of the Placenta: Preliminary Paper," 216; idem, "Further Observations on an Ovary-Stimulating Hormone of the Placenta," 761; idem, "The Ovary Stimulating Hormone of the Placenta," *Nature* 125 (1930): 444.

41 J. Simpson to C.F. Martin, 20 May 1930, RG 38, container 6, file 133, Faculty of Medicine records, MUA.

42 Walter B. Cannon to Isaiah Bowman, 1 February 1935, Walter B. Cannon Papers, box 80, file 1080, Francis Countway Library of Medicine, Harvard Medical School.

43 Jonathan Liebenau, "The MRC and the Pharmaceutical Industry: The Model of Insulin," in *Historical Perspectives on the Role of the MRC*, ed. Joan Austoker and Linda Bryder (Oxford: Oxford University Press 1989), 83–108.

44 In 1943 the foundation was charged with suppressing the use of competing processes, suppressing research data that challenged its financial interests, discouraging firms that held its licences from conducting research, attempting to prevent truthful advertising, and collaborating to maintain artificially high prices for products made under its patents. Charles Weiner, "Patenting and Academic Research: Historical Case Studies," in *Owning Scientific and Technical Information: Values and Ethical Issues*, ed. Vivian Weil and John W. Snapper (New Brunswick, N.J.: Rutgers University Press 1989), 95–9; A. Landsborough Thomson, *Half a Century of Medical Research*, vol. 2: *The Programme of the Medical Research Council (UK)* (London: Her Majesty's Stationery Office 1975), 230–1; Rima D. Apple, "Patenting University Research: Harry Steenbock and the Wisconsin Alumni Research Foundation," *Isis* 80 (1989): 375–94.

45 Walter L. Fletcher to J.B. Collip, 29 April 1930, RG 38, container 6, file 133, Faculty of Medicine records, MUA; MRC memorandum, 1928, quoted in Thomson, *Half a Century of Medical Research* 230–1; Thomson, *Half a Century of Medical Research*, 232.

46 H.H. Dale to J.B. Collip, 30 April 1930, RG 38, container 6, file 133, Faculty of Medicine records, MUA.

47 C.F. Martin to Sir Arthur Currie, 10 May 1930, RG 2, container 66, file 1229, Principal's Papers, MUA.

48 Simpson to C.F. Martin, 11 May 1930, telegram, RG 38, container 6, file 133, Faculty of Medicine records; C.F. Martin to Sir Arthur Currie, 10 May 1930, RG 2, container 66, file 1229, Principal's Papers; and C.F. Martin to Sir Arthur Currie, 13 May 1930, RG 2, container 67, file 1259, Principal's Papers, all in MUA. A.L. Thomson, *Half a Century of Medical Research*, 230.

49 C.F. Martin to Sir Arthur Currie, 13 May 1930, RG 2, container 67, file 1259, Principal's Papers, MUA.

50 J.B. Collip to C.F. Martin, 26 July [1930], RG 38, container 6, file 133, Faculty of Medicine records, MUA.

51 J.B. Collip to C.F. Martin, 26 July [1930], RG 38, container 6, file 133, Faculty of Medicine records, MUA.

52 J.B. Collip to C.F. Martin, 26 July [1930], RG 38, container 6, file 133, Faculty of Medicine records, MUA.

53 Parkes, "The Rise of Reproductive Endocrinology," 33–4.

54 Ibid.

55 J.B. Collip, "The Interrelationship between the Pituitary Gland, the Ovaries and the Placenta," *Transactions of the Royal Society of Canada*, section 5, 26 (1932): 4–5; J.B. Collip, J.S.L. Browne, and D.L. Thomson, "The Relation of Emmenin to Other Estrogenic Hormones," *Journal of Biological Chemistry* 97 (1932): xvii–xviii.

56 C.F. Martin to Sir Ewen Maclean, 6 July 1932, RG 38, container 6, file 133, Faculty of Medicine records, MUA; D.L. Thomson, "Editorial: Emmenin," *Canadian Medical Association Journal* 32 (June 1935): 679–80.

57 W.J. McKenna to C.F. Martin, 1 October 1932, RF 38, container 6, file 133, Faculty of Medicine records, MUA.

58 C.F. Martin to Sir Walter Fletcher, 30 September 1932, unsent, RG 38, container 6, file 133, Faculty of Medicine records, MUA; W. Harrison to Sir Arthur Currie, 30 October 1933, RG 2, container 67, file 1259, Principal's Papers, MUA.

59 W.J. McKenna to C.F. Martin, 1 December 1934, RG 38, container 6, file 133, Faculty of Medicine records, MUA.

60 C.F. Martin to T.C. Routley, 11 December 1934; T.C. Routley to C.F. Martin, 20 December 1934; and Morris Fishbein to R.C. Routley, 8 January 1935, all in RG 38, container 6, file 133, Faculty of Medicine records, MUA.

61 J.C. Simpson to F. Cyril James, 13 December 1940, RG 38, container 6, file 133, Faculty of Medicine records, MUA.

62 There is extensive literature on the tragic consequences of DES use on the children exposed to the drug in utero. DES was widely used until 1970, when it was discovered that daughters with a history of exposure suffered from a rare cancer of the vagina and genital tract abnormalities. See Roberta J. Apfel and Susan M. Fisher, *To Do No Harm: DES and the Dilemmas of Modern Medicine* (New Haven: Yale University Press 1984); and David A. Edelman, *DES/Diethylstilbestrol – New Perspectives* (Lancaster: MTP Press 1986). In a sociological study of the early history of DES (1938–41), Susan Bell examines the role of DES in medicalization of menopause and analyses the interaction among the medical community, the pharmaceutical industry, and government in the development of the drug. Susan E. Bell, "Changing Ideas: The Medicalization of Menopause," *Social Science and Medicine* 24 (1987): 535–42; idem, "A New Model of Medical Technology Development: A Case Study of DES," *Research in the Sociology of Health Care* 4 (1986): 1–32. McGill Board of Governors, Minute No. 214, 28 January 1941, RG 2, container 136, file 3881, Principal's Papers, MUA.

63 *Thirty-Five Years*, 4–6.

64 Alison Li, "Marketing Menopause: Science and the Public Relations of Premarin," in *Women, Health and Nation: Canada and the United States since*

1945, ed. Georgina Feldberg, Molly Ladd-Taylor, Alison Li, and Kathryn McPherson Montreal & Kingston: McGill-Queen's University Press, 2003.

65 J.C. Simpson, Memorandum on Special Funds in the Department of Biochemistry, 19 October 1940, RG 38, container 6, file 133, Faculty of Medicine records, MUA. W.A.S. Ayerst to C.F. Martin, 3 February 1933, and C.F. Martin to Sir Arthur Currie, 4 February 1933, both in RG 2, container 67, file 1259, Principal's Papers, MUA.

66 Vincent Massey to Sir Arthur Currie, 20 January 1933, and Sir Arthur Currie to Vincent Massey, 22 January 1933, both in RG 2, container 67, file 1259, Principal's Papers, MUA.

67 Adele Clarke's use of an industrial model for reproductive science is instructive. She argues that the reproductive research endeavour may truly be termed an enterprise in the sense that research is "a commodity in a marketplace with producers, audiences, sponsors and consumers" and researchers are "entrepreneurs of the enterprise through routine processes of gaining support (fiscal and otherwise) for their work, through publication and so on." Adele E. Clarke, "Emergence of the Reproductive Research Enterprise: A Sociology of Biological Medical and Agricultural Science in the United States" (PhD dissertation, University of California, San Francisco, 1985), 16.

CHAPTER FIVE

1 Fuller Albright and Read Ellsworth, *Uncharted Seas* (Portland, Oreg.: Kalmia Press 1990), 48.

2 J.B. Collip to H.M. Evans, 15 April 1964, H.M. Evans Papers, carton 2, box 17, University of California, Berkeley Archives.

3 D.L. Thomson, "Dr. James Bertram Collip," *Canadian Journal of Biochemistry and Physiology* 35, suppl. (1957): 3–7; R.L. Noble, "Memories of James Bertram Collip," *Canadian Medical Association Journal* 93 (1965): 1356–64.

4 D.L. Thomson, "Dr. James Bertram Collip," 6; J.S.L. Browne and O.F. Denstedt, "James Bertram Collip (1892–1965)," *Endocrinology* 79 (1966): 225–8; interview with Dr A.E. Neufeld by author, 18 October 1993. None of Collip's little black notebooks survive to my knowledge, except for the one page detailing the method of making insulin. Collip's procedure for extracting insulin, 22 December 1921, MS Collection 269, item 1, Fisher Rare Book Library, UT.

5 D.K. O'Donovan, "Some Reminiscences of Canadian Endocrinology," *Journal of the Irish Medical Association* 69 (1976): 298–9; Browne and Denstedt, "James Bertram Collip," 228.

6 Browne and Denstedt, "James Bertram Collip," 228; A. Neufeld, "Comments by Abe Neufeld re: Dr. J.B. Collip," file "Library," Collip

Correspondence, Regional Collection, University of Western Ontario, 2–3; interview with Dr A.E. Neufeld by author, 18 October 1993.

7 Interview with Drs Barbara and C.J. Wyatt, 11 February 1995, by author.

8 Browne and Denstedt, "James Bertram Collip," 228; Thomson, "Dr. James Bertram Collip," 4–5; A. Neufeld, "Comments by Abe Neufeld re: Dr. J.B. Collip," file "Library," Collip Correspondence, Regional Collection, uwo, 3; Warren Weaver diary, 9 February 1934, RF, RG 2, series 427D, box 103, folder 808, RAC.

9 Hans Selye, *The Stress of My Life*, 2nd ed. (New York: Van Nostrand Reinhold 1979), 47–52; Frank Blair Hanson diary, 9 February 1934, RF, RG 2, series 427D, box 103, folder 808, RAC.

10 Noble, "Memories," 1360–1; R.J. Rossiter, "James Bertram Collip, 1892–1965," *Proceedings and Transactions of the Royal Society of Canada* 4 (1966): 73–82; Browne and Denstedt, "James Bertram Collip," 228; Thomson, "Dr. James Bertram Collip," 6.

11 Interview with Drs Barbara and C.J. Wyatt, 11 February 1995, by author.

12 M.K. McPhail, typescript beginning "the impressions that I have of Dr. Collip," Collip Papers, Regional Collection, uwo; Noble, "Memories," 1360; Browne and Denstedt, "James Bertram Collip," 28; interview with Drs Barbara and C.J. Wyatt, 11 February 1995, by author.

13 Bensley, *McGill Medical Luminaries*, 111–12.

14 After he retired at McGill, Murray took up Collip's offer of a guest professorship at the University of Western Ontario. C.E. Dolman, "Everitt George Dunne Murray, 1890–1964," *Proceedings of the Royal Society of Canada* 3, series 4 (1965): 145–53; David A. Keys, "James Bertram Collip, An Appreciation," *Canadian Medical Association Journal* 93 (1965): 774–5.

15 D. Sclater Lewis, *Royal Victoria Hospital, 1887–1947* (Montreal: McGill University Press 1969), 169–79.

16 I.M. Rabinowitch to O.R. Denstedt, 10 March 1969, AC 2049, MG 1031, O.F. Denstedt Papers, MUA; Bensley, *McGill Medical Luminaries*, 139–40.

17 J.B. Collip, D.L. Thomson, M.K. McPhail, and J.E. Williamson, "The Anterior-Pituitary-Like Hormone of the Human Placenta," *Canadian Medical Association Journal* 24 (1931): 201–10.

18 Diana Long Hall and Thomas Glick, "Endocrinology: A Brief Introduction," *Journal of the History of Biology* 9 (1976): 229–33. The field of reproductive endocrinology was opened by the isolation of estrin. This was the work of the biochemist Edward Doisy and the zoologist Edgar Allen, who began their successful collaboration after meeting on a faculty baseball team. Medvei, *A History of Endocrinology*, 397–8.

19 Charles H. Sawyer, "Anterior Pituitary Neural Control Concepts," in *Endocrinology: People and Ideas*, ed. S.M. McCann (Bethesda, Md.: American Physiological Society, 1988), 26; E.C. Amoroso and G.W. Cor-

ner, "Herbert McLean Evans," *Biographical Memoirs of Fellows of the Royal Society* 18 (1972): 122–4; Medvei, *A History of Endocrinology,* 315, 518–19.

20 Adele Clarke, "Research Materials and Reproductive Science in the United States, 1910–1940," in *Physiology in the American Context, 1850–1940,* ed. Gerald L. Geison (Bethesda, Md.: American Physiological Society 1987), 323–50; W. Lane-Petter, "The Experimental Animal in Research," *Techniques in Endocrine Research,* ed. Peter Eckstein and Francis Knowles (London: Academic Press 1963), 149–59.

21 J.B. Collip, H. Selye, and D.L. Thomson, "Gonad-Stimulating Hormones in Hypophysectomized Animals," *Nature* 131 (1933): 56; J.B. Collip, "The Anterior Pituitary Lobe: Fractionation of Active Principle," *Lancet* 224 (1933): 1208; Frank Blair Hanson, 9 February 1934, RG 2, series 427D, box 103, folder 808, RAC; J.B. Collip, "Report to the Dean of the Research Work in the Department of Biochemistry during the Current Year – 1932," RG 2, container 67, file 1258, Principal's Papers, MUA.

22 O.F. Denstedt, "The Evolution of Biochemistry at McGill," typescript, MG 1031, O.F. Denstedt Papers, MUA, 10–13; Frank Blair Hanson, 9 February 1934, RG 2, series 427D, box 103, folder 808, RAC; J.B. Collip, Hans Selye, Evelyn M. Anderson, and D.L. Thomson, "Production of Estrus: Relationship between Active Principles of the Placenta and Pregnancy Blood and Urine and Those of the Anterior Pituitary," *Journal of the American Medical Association* 1010 (1933): 1553.

23 J.B. Collip, "Chemistry and Physiology of Anterior Pituitary Hormones," *Transactions of the Congress of American Physicians and Surgeons* 15 (1933): 47–64.

24 E.M. Anderson and J.B. Collip, "Thyreotropic Hormone of Anterior Pituitary," *Proceedings of the Society for Experimental Biology and Medicine* 30 (1933): 680–3; Evelyn M. Anderson and J.B. Collip, "Studies on the Physiology of the Thyreotropic Hormone of the Anterior Pituitary," *Journal of Physiology* 82 (1934): 11–25; J.B. Collip, Evelyn M. Anderson, and D.L. Thomson, "The Adrenotropic Hormone of the Anterior Pituitary Lobe," *Lancet* 225 (1933): 347–8; Choh Hao Li, Herbert M. Evans, and Miriam E. Simpson, "Adrenocorticotropic Hormone," *Journal of Biological Chemistry* 149 (1943): 413–24; George Sayers, Abraham White, and C.N.H. Long, "Preparation and Properties of Pituitary Adrenotropic Hormone," *Journal of Biological Chemistry* 149 (1943): 425–36.

25 Interview with Drs Barbara and C.J. Wyatt, 11 February 1995, by author.

26 Noble, "Memories," 1364.

27 Medvei, *A History of Endocrinology,* 520–4; Amoroso and Corner, "Herbert McLean Evans," 100–1.

28 Amoroso and Corner, "Herbert McLean Evans," 83–186.

29 Interview with Dr A.E. Neufeld, 18 October 1993, by author.
30 Interview with R.L. Noble, Vancouver, B.C., 5 June 1990, by author, notes; Warren Weaver diary, 25 January 1937, RG 2, series 427D, box 150, folder 110, RAC; J.B. Collip, H. Selye, and D.L. Thomson, "Beiträge zur Kenntnis der Physiologie des Gehirnanhanges," *Virchows Archiv für Pathologishe Anatomie und Physiologie* 290 (1933): 23–46.
31 J.B. Collip, discussion in "Panel Discussion on the Pituitary Gland," *Journal of Pediatrics* 8 (1936): 393.
32 J.B. Collip, "The Anterior Pituitary Lobe: Fractionation of Active Principle," *Lancet* 224 (1933): 1209.
33 Herbert M. Evans, "Present Position of Our Knowledge of Anterior Pituitary Function," *Journal of the American Medical Association* 101 (1933): 426, 432.
34 Warren Weaver diary, 25 January 1937, RG 2, series 427D, box 150, folder 110, RAC.
35 J.B. Collip, "Inhibitory Hormones and the Principle of Inverse Response," *Annals of Internal Medicine* 8 (1934): 10–13; Garland Allen, *Life Science in the Twentieth Century* (Cambridge: Cambridge University Press 1975), 95–103.
36 Evelyn M. Anderson and J.B. Collip, "Preparation and Properties of an Antithyrotropic Substance," *Lancet* 226 (1934): 784–6; C. Bachman, J.B. Collip, and H. Selye, "Anti-Gonadotropic Substances," *Proceedings of the Society for Experimental Biology and Medicine* 32 (1934): 544–7; R.G. Hoskins, discussion in "Panel Discussion on the Pituitary Gland," *Journal of Pediatrics* 8 (1936): 399.
37 J.B. Collip and Evelyn M. Anderson, "Studies on the Thyreotropic Hormone of the Anterior Pituitary," *Journal of the American Medical Association* 104 (1935): 965–9; J.B. Collip, H. Selye, and J.E. Williamson, "Changes in the Hypophysis and the Ovaries of Rats Chronically Treated with an Anterior Pituitary Extract," *Endocrinology* 23 (1938): 279–84.
38 Selye, *Stress of My Life*, 59–62; H. Selye and J.B. Collip, "Fundamental Factors in the Interpretation of Stimuli Influencing Endocrine Glands," *Endocrinology* 20 (1936): 667–72.
39 There is a long-standing and widespread opinion that this parting of ways was very bitter and that Collip's poor opinion of Selye's work continued for many years. However, Selye's work inspired the confidence of C.P. Martin, the head of the Department of Anatomy, Histology, and Embryology, and G. Fleming, the dean of medicine. They endeavoured to secure Selye funding from the Carnegie Institute to allow him to carry out his work. Selye remained in the Department of Anatomy teaching histology and taking charge of graduate research until 1945. He admitted that he had always preferred hormone research to teaching histology and longed to have an independent institute or department devoted to endocrine research, but as

Collip's institute had been created by that time, this was not possible at
McGill. Selye accepted the directorship of the Institute of Experimental
Medicine and Surgery at the University of Montreal. C.P. Martin to J.C.
Simpson, 17 April 1938; G. Fleming to L.W. Douglas, 22 April 1938; and
H. Selye to F. Cyril James, 30 August 1945, all in RG 39, container 6,
file 130, Faculty of Medicine records, MUA.

40 Hans Selye, "Adaptation to Oestrogen Overdosage: An Acquired Hormone
Resistance without Antihormone Formation," *American Journal of Physiology* 30 (1940): 258–64; idem, "The General Adaptation Syndrome and the
Diseases of Adaptation," *Journal of Clinical Endocrinology* 6 (1946): 117–
230.

41 J.B. Collip, "Results of Recent Studies on Anterior Pituitary Hormones,"
Edinburgh Medical Journal 45 (1938): 801; David L. Thomson, James B.
Collip, and Hans Selye, "The Antihormones," *Journal of the American
Medical Association* 116 (1941): 132–6.

42 H.M. Evans, discussion in James H. Leathem, "The Antihormone Problem
in Endocrine Therapy," *Recent Progress in Hormone Research* 4 (1949):
143. Later work provided unequivocal evidence that even completely pure
hormone preparations are capable of raising antibodies. Roy O. Greep,
"Gonadotropins," in *Endocrinology: People and Ideas*, ed. S.M. McCann
(Bethesda, Md: American Physiological Society 1988), 82.

43 Greep, "Gonadotropins," 80–2; Noble, "Memories," 1360; D.L. Thomson, "Dr. James Bertram Collip," 5.

44 Schwartz, "Giants with Tunnel Vision," 327–46.

45 Fuller Albright to J.B. Collip, 11 April 1940, and J.B. Collip to Fuller Albright, 19 April 1940, both in box 11, file "C inactive," Fuller Albright Papers, Francis Countway Library, Harvard Medical School; Christiane
Sinding, "Clinical Research and Basic Science: The Development of the
Concept of End-Organ Resistance to a Hormone," *Journal of the History
of Medicine and Allied Sciences* 45 (1990): 198–232.

46 J.B. Collip, "Demonstration of an Orally Active Medullotrophic Principle
in a Primary Extract of Pituitary Tissue," *Canadian Medical Association
Journal* 42 (1940): 2–4; A.H. Neufeld and J.B. Collip, "Studies of the Ef-
fects of Pituitary Extracts on Carbohydrate and Fat Metabolism," *Endocri-
nology* 23 (1938): 735–46; D.K. O'Donovan and J.B. Collip, "The Specific
Metabolic Principle of the Pituitary and Its Relation to the Melanophore
Hormone," *Endocrinology* 23 (1938): 718–34; Noble, "Memories," 1361;
I.M. Rabinowitch, Marjorie Mountford, D.K. O'Donovan, and J.B. Collip,
"Influence of a Specific Hormone of the Pituitary on the Basal Metabolism
in Man," *Canadian Medical Association Journal* 40 (1939): 105–7.

47 R.L. Noble, C.S. McEuen, and J.B. Collip, "Mammary Tumours Produced
in Rats by the Action of Oestrone Tablets," *Canadian Medical Association
Journal* 42 (1940): 413–17; R.L. Noble and J.B. Collip, "A Quantitative

Method for the Production of Experimental Traumatic Shock without Haemorrhage in Unanesthetized Animals," *Quarterly Journal of Experimental Physiology* 13 (1942): 187–99.

48 Choh Hao Li, Herbert M. Evans, and Miriam E. Simpson, "Adrenocorticotropic Hormone," *Journal of Biological Chemistry* 149 (1943): 413; Walter Marx, Miriam E. Simpson, and Herbert M. Evans, "Bioassay of the Growth Hormone of the Anterior Pituitary," *Endocrinology* 30 (1942): 1–10; Amoroso and Corner, "Herbert McLean Evans," 122.

49 Noble, "Memories," 1363.

50 E. Gordon Young, *The Development of Biochemistry in Canada* (Toronto: University of Toronto Press 1976), 104–7.

51 J.B. Collip to H.M. Evans, 15 April 1964, H.M. Evans Papers, carton 2, box 17, University of California, Berkeley Archives.

52 This point is examined in greater depth in the following chapter.

CHAPTER SIX

1 J.B. Collip to C.F. Martin, 15 December 1934, RF, RG 2, series 427D, box 103, folder 808, RAC.

2 Gina Feldberg, "The Origins of Organized Canadian Medical Research: The National Research Council's Association Committee on Tuberculosis Research," *Scientia Canadensis* 15, no. 2 (1991): 53–69. The University of Manitoba and Queen's University awarded eight and six PhDs respectively during the period from 1920 to 1940. Robin S. Harris, *A History of Higher Education in Canada, 1663–1960* (Toronto: University of Toronto Press 1976), 431.

3 Stanley Brice Frost, *McGill University for the Advancement of Learning*, vol. 2: *1895–1971* (Montreal & Kingston: McGill-Queen's University Press 1984), 188.

4 Bensley, *McGill Medical Luminaries*, 122–5; Frost, *McGill University*, 164–73; *McGill University Annual Report, 1933–34*, 22.

5 Frank Blair Hanson diary, 9 February 1934, RF, RG 2, series 427D, box 103, folder 808, RAC.

6 Bliss, *Discovery of Insulin*, 240–1; "Department of Biochemistry Statement of Income & Expenditure from June 1, 1931 to May 31, 1935 with Estimated Figures for Year Ending May 31, 1936," RG 2, container 67, file 1262, Principal's Papers, MUA. The Rockefeller Foundation endowments had been set up to yield higher incomes, but during the Depression there was a steady depreciation of the interest. The Montreal Neurological Institute endowment was intended to bring $50,000 a year. "Research Funds in the Medical Faculty," 1 October 1935, RG 2, container 66, file 1244, Principal's Papers, MUA; J.C. Meakins to Allen Greig [Alan Gregg], 2 September 1937, RF, RG 1.1, series 427A, box 6, folder 49, RAC.

7 F. Owen Stredder to J.C. Simpson, 29 January 1937; and "Memorandum on Special Funds in the Department of Biochemistry, submitted by the dean of the Faculty of Medicine," 19 October 1940, both in RG 38, container 6, file 133, Faculty of Medicine records, MUA. The Premarin royalty figure is based on an estimate from royalties of $13,287 over a three-month period. G.S. McFadden to F. Cyril James, 19 August 1947, RG 2, container 136, file 3881, Principal's Papers, MUA; F. Cyril James to J.B. Collip, 6 August 1941, MS Collection 269, item 3, Collip Papers, Fisher Rare Book Library, UT. To help the reader gauge these sums, it may help to know that Collip's salary as professor was $8,100 in 1937 and that when he was appointed dean of medicine at the University of Western Ontario, it was at a salary of $10,000. J.C. Simpson to W.H. Brittain, 5 October 1937, RG 38, container 6, file 133, Faculty of Medicine records, MUA; G.E. Hall to J.B. Collip, 16 April 1947, Collip Papers, Regional Collection, UWO.

8 "Department of Biochemistry Statement of Income & Expenditure from June 1, 1931 to May 31, 1935 with Estimated Figures for Year Ending May 31, 1936," RG 2, container 67, file 1262, Principal's Papers, MUA.

9 Claude Bissell, *The Young Vincent Massey* (Toronto: University of Toronto Press 1981), 157; Vincent Massey to Arthur Currie, 20 January 1933, RG 2, container 67, file 1259, Principal's Papers, MUA; Vincent Massey to J.B. Collip, 22 December 1934, MS Collection 269, item 3, Collip Papers, Fisher Rare Book Library, UT.

10 Robert Kohler, *Partners in Science* (Chicago: University of Chicago Press 1991), 233–62, 265–83.

11 R.M. Pierce to G.A. Brakeley, 25 February 1929, RF, RG 2, series 427D, box 103, folder 808, RAC.

12 Frank Blair Hanson diary, 9 February 1934, and Warren Weaver diary, 9 February 1934, both in RF, RG 2, series 427D, box 103, folder 808, RAC.

13 Warren Weaver diary, 9 February 1934, RF, RG 2, series 427D, box 103, folder 808, RAC. After 1930 the Banting and Best department was located on one floor of the Banting Institute building. The institute had no real existence as such, and this was a source of great confusion. Bliss, *Discovery of Insulin*, 235.

14 Warren Weaver diary, 27 February 1934, RF, RG 2, series 427D, box 103, folder 808, RAC.

15 C.F. Martin to Warren Weaver, 9 March 1934, and Warren Weaver diary, 29 March 1934, both in RF, RG 2, series 427D, box 103, folder 808, RAC.

16 J.B. Collip to C.F. Martin, 15 December 1934, RF, RG 2, series 427D, box 103, folder 808, RAC.

17 J.B. Collip to C.F. Martin, 15 December 1934, RF, RG 2, series 427D, box 103, folder 808, RAC.

18 J.B. Collip to C.F. Martin, 15 December 1934, RF, RG 2, series 427D, box 103, folder 808, RAC.

19 C.F. Martin to Alan Gregg, 8 January 1935, and Warren Weaver diary, 19 March 1935, both in RF, RG 2, series 427D, box 121, folder 919, RAC.

20 Warren Weaver diary, 19 March 1935, RG, RG 2, series 427D, box 121, folder 919, RAC.

21 Warren Weaver diary, 19 March 1935, and Alan Gregg diary, 19 March 1935, both in RF, RG 2, series 427D, box 121, folder 919, RAC.

22 P.W. MacFarlane to C.F. Martin, 24 March 1935, RF, RG 2, container 67, file 1262, MUA; C.F. Martin to Warren Weaver, 23 March 1935, RF, RG 2, series 427D, box 121, folder 919, RAC.

23 C.F. Martin to Warren Weaver, 23 March 1935, RF, RG 2, series 427D, box 121, folder 919, RAC.

24 J.B. Collip to C.F. Martin, 23 March 1935, and C.F. Martin to Warren Weaver, 23 March 1935, both in RF, RG 2, series 427D, box 121, folder 919, RAC.

25 Warren Weaver, inter-office correspondence, 27 March 1935, and Warren Weaver to C.F. Martin, 15 April 1935, both in RF, RG 2, series 427D, box 121, folder 919, RAC.

26 J.B. Collip to William Rowan, 18 June 1935, 69–16–181, William Rowan Papers, UAA.

27 C.F. Martin to Warren Weaver, 27 August 1935, and Warren Weaver diary, 9 September 1935, both in RF, RG 2, series 427D, box 121, folder 919, RAC.

28 Warren Weaver diary, 9 September 1935, RF, RG 2, series 427D, box 121, folder 919, RAC.

29 Warren Weaver to C.F. Martin, 19 September 1935, and C.F. Martin to Warren Weaver, 23 September 1935, both in RF, RG 2, series 427D, box 121, folder 919, RAC.

30 Harry M. Miller diary, 26 October 1935, RF, RG 2, series 427D, box 121, folder 919, RAC.

31 Frost, *McGill University*, 192.

32 Ibid., 190.

33 Arthur E. Morgan to Warren Weaver, 13 December 1935, RG 2, container 67, file 1262, Principal's Papers, MUA.

34 Warren Weaver diary, 17 December 1935, RF, RG 2, series 427D, box 121, folder 919, RAC.

35 "The Principal's Memorandum of his interview with Dr. Warren Weaver. December 17th, at the Rockefeller Foundation Offices," 18 December 1935, RG 2, container 67, file 1262, Principal's Papers, MUA; Warren Weaver diary, 17 December 1935, RF, RG 2, series 427D, box 121, folder 919, RAC.

36 "The Principal's Memorandum of his interview with Dr. Warren Weaver. December 17th, at the Rockefeller Foundation Offices," 18 December 1935, RG 2, container 67, file 1262, Principal's Papers, MUA.

37 Warren Weaver diary, 17 December 1935, RF, RG 2, series 427D, box 121, folder 919, RAC.

38 A.E. Morgan to Warren Weaver, 18 December 1935, RG 2, container 67, file 1262, Principal's Papers, MUA; Frost, *McGill University*, 190–7; *McGill University Annual Report*, 1935–6.

39 J.B. Collip, "Hormones in Relation to Human Behavior," in Harvard Tercentenary Conference of Arts and Sciences, *Factors Determining Human Behavior* (Cambridge, Mass.: Harvard University Press 1937), 12–31.

40 J.B. Collip to William Rowan, 12 November 1942, 69–16–181, William Rowan Papers, UAA; Ainley, *Restless Energy*, 139, 168, 171.

41 Frank Blair Hanson diary, 7 and 8 September 1936, RF, RG 2, series 427D, box 121, folder 919; and Warren Weaver, 12 January 1937, RF, RG 2, series 427D, box 150, folder 1110, both in RAC.

42 Wilder Penfield, *The Difficult Art of Giving: The Epic of Alan Gregg* (Boston, Toronto: Little, Brown and Company 1967), 230–50; Raymond B. Fosdick, foreword in *The Difficult Art of Giving*, x–xi; Kohler, *Partners in Science*, 401–2.

43 *Rockefeller Foundation Report*, 1935, 163; *Rockefeller Foundation Report*, 1936, 197.

44 Kohler, *Partners in Science*, 398.

45 Warren Weaver, inter-office correspondence, 18 September 1937, RF, RG 1.1, series 427A, box 6, folder 49, RAC.

46 "The Principal's Private Memorandum for the File," 9 April 1937, RG 2, container 67, file 1262, Principal's Papers, MUA.

47 *McGill University Annual Report, 1936–1937*, 28; A.E. Morgan to J.B. Collip, 15 April 1937, RG 2, container 67, file 1262, Principal's Papers, MUA.

48 J.B. Collip to A.E. Morgan, 15 April 1937, RG 2, container 67, file 1262, Principal's Papers, MUA.

49 J.B. Collip to A.E. Morgan, 15 April 1937, RG 2, container 67, file 1262, Principal's Papers, MUA.

50 Frost, *McGill University*, 190–7.

51 J.C. Simpson to W.H. Brittain, 5 October 1937, RG 38, container 6, file 133, Faculty of Medicine records, MUA.

52 Interview with Drs Barbara and C.J. Wyatt, 11 February 1995, by author.

53 F. Owen Stredder to J.B. Collip, 21 October 1937, RG 38, container 6, file 133, Faculty of Medicine records; "James B. Collip Mortgage – 622 Sydenham Ave. Westmount," RG 2, container 136, file 3881, Principal's Papers; and "Memorandum on Special Funds in the Department of Biochemistry submitted by the Dean of the Faculty of Medicine," 19 October 1940, RG 38, container 6, file 133, Faculty of Medicine records, all in MUA.

54 Donald Avery, *The Science of War: Canadian Scientists and Allied Military Technology during the Second World War* (Toronto: University of Toronto Press 1998).

55 Frank Blair Hanson interview, 15 May 1940, RF, RG 2, series 427D, box 201, folder 1421, RAC.

56 For example, the MNI received a donation of $50,000 in 1930 from Madeleine Ottman. *McGill University Annual Report, 1930–1931*. L.W. Douglas to Sir Herbert Holt, 7 October 1938, RG 2, container 55, file 783, Principal's Papers; Herbert S. Holt to Lewis W. Douglas, 11 October 1938, RG 2, container 55, file 783, Principal's Papers; L.W. Douglas to Sir Herbert Holt, 12 October 1938, RG 2, container 55, file 783, Principal's Papers; "Memorandum on Special Funds in the Department of Biochemistry, submitted by the Dean of the Faculty of Medicine," 19 October 1940, RG 38, container 6, file 133, Faculty of Medicine records; F. Owen Stredder to L.W. Douglas, 25 October 1938, RG 2, container 55, file 783, Principal's Papers; F. Owen Stredder to L.W. Douglas, 28 October 1938, RG 2, container 55, file 783, Principal's Papers, all in MUA.

57 "Memorandum on Special Funds in the Department of Biochemistry, submitted by the Dean of the Faculty of Medicine," 19 October 1940, RF 38, container 6, file 133, Faculty of Medicine records, MUA; F. Lorne Hutchison to J.B. Collip, 3 July 1948, Collip Papers, Regional Collection, UWO; Young, *The Development of Biochemistry in Canada*, 52–3; Bliss, *Discovery of Insulin*, 240. F. Lorne Hutchison to J.B. Collip, 20 June 1950; Eugene Beesley to J.B. Collip, 8 February 1955; and Ewald Rohrmann to J.B. Collip, 18 October 1956, all in Collip Papers, Regional Collection, UWO. Swann, *Academic Scientists and the Pharmaceutical Industry*, 148–9.

58 Frost, *McGill University*, 214; ibid., 205–16.

59 Bliss, *Banting, A Biography*, 288–90; idem, "Rewriting Medical History: Charles Best and the Banting and Best Myth," *Journal of the History of Medicine and Allied Sciences* 48, no. 3 (1993): 253–74.

60 Bliss, *Banting, A Biography*, 300–7.

61 George Hunter to J.B. Collip, 27 February 1941, Collip Papers, Regional Collection, UWO.

62 Saide Gairns to J.B. Collip, 14 June 1941, MS Collection 269, item 2, Collip Papers, Fisher Rare Book Library, UT.

63 F. Cyril James to F.C. MacIntosh, 20 October 1965, "Library" file, Collip Correspondence, Regional Collection, UWO.

64 F. Cyril James to F.C. MacIntosh, 20 October 1965, "Library" file, Collip Correspondence, Regional Collection, UWO.

65 F. Cyril James to J.B. Collip, 6 August 1941, MS Collection 169, item 3, Collip Papers, Fisher Rare Book Library, UT.

66 R.S. Morison interview, 6 March 1946, RF, RG 2, series 427D, box 344, folder 2328, RAC.

67 Orville F. Denstedt, "The Evolution of Biochemistry at McGill," O.F. Denstedt Papers, MG 1031, MUA, 13; Orville Denstedt to G. Lyman Duff, 6 January 1950, RG 2, container 136, file 3872, Principal's Papers, MUA.

68 J.B. Collip, manuscript of speech upon leaving McGill in 1947, MS Collection 269, item 4, Collip Papers, Fisher Rare Book Library, UT.

69 F. Cyril James to J.B. Collip, 7 July 1942, MS Collection 269, item 4, Collip Papers, Fisher Rare Book Library, UT.

70 *Proceedings of the Conference on Motion Sickness Held Jointly under the Associate Committee on Medical Research and Associate Committee on Aviation Medical Research*, 28 August 1942, Records Office, NRC.

71 G.H. Ettinger, *History of the Associate Committee on Medical Research* (Ottawa: National Research Council 1946), 20.

72 *Proceedings of the Sixth Meeting of the Associate Committee on Army Medical Research*, vol. 11, Addenda, Records Office, NRC.

73 R.S. Morison interview, 6 March 1946, RF, RG 2, series 427D, box 344, folder 2328; and R.S. Morison to Warren Weaver, 6 May 1946, RF, RG 2, series 427D, box 344, folder 2328, both at RAC.

74 Michael R. Marrus, *Mr Sam: The Life and Times of Samuel Bronfman* (Toronto: Viking 1991), 299, 411–12.

75 F. Cyril James to J.B. Collip, 23 December 1946, and F. Cyril James to Allan Bronfman, 13 March 1947, both in RG 2, container 136, file 3881, Principal's Papers, MUA. Interview with R.L. Noble, 4 June 1990, Vancouver, B.C., by author.

76 G.E. Hall to J.B. Collip, 24 December 1943, MS Collection 269, item 4, Collip Papers, Fisher Rare Book Library, UT.

77 R.S. Morison interview, 6 March 1946, RF, RG 2, series 427D, box 344, folder 2328, RAC; J.B. Collip, Addison Lecture, July 1948, MS Collection 269, item 4, Collip Papers, Fisher Rare Book Library, UT.

78 J.B. Collip and Ray Collip to Dr and Mrs C.F. Martin, undated [April 1947?], MS Collection 269, item 4, Collip Papers, Fisher Rare Book Library, UT.

79 J.B. Collip to F. Cyril James, 15 March 1947, RG 2, container 136, file 3881, Principal's Papers, MUA; G.E. Hall to J.B. Collip, 5 April 1947, Collip Papers, Regional Collection, UWO; F. Cyril James to J.B. Collip, 14 April 1947, RG 2, container 136, file 3881, Principal's Papers, MUA.

80 G.E. Hall to the Council of the Faculty of Medicine, 15 April 1947, file 1, Collip Correspondence, Regional Collection, UWO; F. Cyril James to W. Sherwood Fox, 18 April 1947, RG 2, container 136, file 3881, Principal's Papers, MUA.

81 Stanley Brice Frost, *The Man in the Ivory Tower: F. Cyril James of McGill* (Montreal & Kingston: McGill-Queen's University Press 1991), 154; F. Cyril James to W.W. Chipman, 24 April 1947, RG 2, container 136, file 3881, Principal's Papers, MUA; R.B. Willis to J.B. Collip, 8 July 1947, Collip Papers, Regional Collection, UWO. Insulin Fund, $42,208; Emmenin Fund, $136,111; Premarin Fund, $119,458; Pituitrin Fund, $4,992, for a total of $743,440. "McGill University Summary Statement of

Endocrinology Royalty Funds at March 31, 1947," RG 2, container 136, file 3881, Principal's Papers, MUA.

82 F. Cyril James to W.W. Chipman, 24 April 1947, RG 2, container 136, file 3881, Principal's Papers, MUA.

83 J.B. Collip and Ray Collip to Dr and Mrs C.F. Martin, undated [April 1947?], MS Collection 269, item 4, Collip Papers, Fisher Rare Book Library, UT.

84 Harold Ettinger to J.B. Collip, 22 April 1947; C.J. Mackenzie to J.B. Collip, 26 April 1947; J.A. Gray to J.B. Collip, 29 April 1947; C. Leonard Huskins, undated [May 1947?]; L. Austin Wright, 23 April 1947; J.B. Collip to Charles A. Mitchell, 3 May 1947; Charles A. Mitchell to J.B. Collip, 28 April 1947, all in MS Collection 269, item 4, Collip Papers, Fisher Rare Book Library, UT.

85 J.B. Collip to F. Cyril James, 26 July 1947, RG 2, container 136, file 3881, Principal's Papers, MUA. McGill received $10,000, while UWO received $25,000. William Bentley to F. Cyril James, 17 May 1947, RG 2, container 136, file 3881, Principal's Papers, MUA; memorandum of agreement between McGill University and Ayerst, McKenna & Harrison Ltd, 1 July 1947, RG 2, container 136, file 3881, Principal's Papers, MUA; W.A. Leslie to G.E. Hall, 29 July 1947, P3, Medical Research, President's file, Regional Collection, UWO; D.L. Thomson to F. Cyril James, 7 June 1947, RF 38, container 6, file 133, Faculty of Medicine records, MUA; D.L. Thomson to F. Cyril James, 18 November 1947, RF 2, container 136, file 3874, Principal's Papers, MUA.

86 F. Cyril James to F.C. MacIntosh, 20 October 1965, "Library" file, Collip Correspondence, Regional Collection, UWO.

CHAPTER SEVEN

1 *Proceedings of the Conference on the Organization of Medical Research in Canada*, 18 February 1938, 11, Records Office, NRC.

2 M.L. Barr and R.J. Rossiter, "James Bertram Collip, 1892–1965," *Biographical Memoirs of Fellows of the Royal Society* 19 (1973): 249–50.

3 Alison Li, "Expansion and Consolidation: The Associate Committee and the Division of Medical Research of the National Research Council," *Scientia Canadensis* 15, no. 2 (1990): 89–104.

4 Frederick Banting and C.B. Stewart, *Survey of Facilities for Medical Research in Canada* (Ottawa: National Research Council 1939).

5 In Great Britain, the Medical Research Committee was established in 1913 and succeeded by the Medical Research Council in 1920. The council employed technical and scientific staff at its research units at medical schools and hospitals and at its central research establishment, the National Institute for Medical Research at Mill Hill. In the United States, the Public

Health Service established its national research centre, the National Institutes of Health, in Bethesda, Maryland, in 1930. C.B. Stewart, "Reminiscences on the Founding and Early History of the Medical Research Council of Canada: Part 2," *Annals of the Royal College of Physicians and Surgeons of Canada* 9 (1986): 473.

6 Richard A. Jarrell and Yves Gingras, eds, *Building Canadian Science: The Role of the National Research Council* (Ottawa: Canadian Science and Technology Historical Association 1992), special no. of *Scientia Canadensis* 15, no. 2 (1991); Yves Gingras, "Financial Support for Post-graduate Students and the Development of Scientific Research in Canada," in *Youth, University and Canadian Society: Essays in the Social History of Higher Education*, ed. Paul Axelrod and John G. Reid (Montreal & Kingston: McGill-Queen's University Press 1989), 301–19; Georgina Feldberg, "The Origins of Organized Canadian Medical Research: The National Research Council's Associate Committee on Tuberculosis Research, 1924–1938," *Scientia Canadensis* 15, no. 2 (1991): 53–69; Wilfrid Eggleston, *National Research in Canada: The NRC 1916–1966* (Toronto: Clarke Irwin 1978), 339. Macallum was an influential advocate of pure research at universities and of the creation of a central NRC laboratory for industrial research. Philip C. Enros, "'The Onery Council of Scientific and Industrial Pretence': Universities and the Early NRC's Plans for Industrial Research," *Scientia Canadensis* 14, no. 2 (1991): 41–51.

7 Harris, *History of Higher Education*, 320.

8 Bliss, *Discovery of Insulin*, 240.

9 G.H. Ettinger, "The Origins of Support for Medical Research in Canada," *Canadian Medical Association Journal* 78 (1958): 471; "The Organization of Medical Research in Canada," draft proposal, 23 November 1936, Banting Papers, Canadian Institute for Scientific and Technical Information (hereafter CISTI); A.G. McNaughton, "Memorandum reporting conversations and discussions on the subject of the proposed organization of an Associate Committee on Medical Research," 8 September 1937–11 September 1937, Banting Papers, CISTI; *Proceedings of the Second Meeting of the Preparatory Committee*, 18 December 1937, 5, Records Office, NRC.

10 A. Landsborough Thomson, *Half a Century of Medical Research*, vols 1 and 2 (London: Her Majesty's Stationery Office, 1973, 1975); Joan Austoker and Linda Bryder, eds, *Historical Perspectives on the Role of the MRC* (Oxford: Oxford University Press 1989); A.T. Bazin, "Report of Committee on Organization of Medical Research in Canada," undated, Banting Papers, CISTI; McNaughton, "Memorandum reporting conversations and discussions."

11 J.G. FitzGerald to A.G.L. McNaughton, 9 November 1937, Banting Papers, CISTI.

12 *Proceedings of the Conference on the Organization of Medical Research in Canada*, 18 February 1938, 11, Records Office, NRC.

13 *Organization of Medical Research in Canada: Proceedings of a Preliminary Conference*, 28 October 1937, 4–5, Records Office, NRC; *Proceedings of the Conference on the Organization*, 21–2.

14 *Proceedings of the Conference on the Organization*, 33.

15 Ibid., 43, app. 5.

16 Banting and Stewart, *Survey of Facilities*; Stewart, "Reminiscences," 388; G.H. Ettinger, "Medical Research," in *Royal Commission Studies: A Selection of Essays Prepared for the Royal Commission on National Development in the Arts, Letters, and Sciences* (Ottawa: Edmond Cloutier 1951), 317–36.

17 F.G. Banting to Wilder Penfield, 1 February 1939, Banting Papers, CISTI.

18 Proceedings of the First Meeting of the Associate Committee on Medical Research, 6 May 1938, 21, Records Office, NRC; Proceedings of the Third Meeting of the Associate Committee on Medical Research, 27–28 February 1939, 8, Records Office, NRC.

19 Harris, *History of Higher Education*, 563–4.

20 Banting and Collip had become estranged from Best in later years. For information on the wartime committees and the roles of Banting, Best, and Collip, see Terrie M. Romano, "The Associate Committees on Medical Research of the National Research Council and the Second World War," *Scientia Canadensis* 15, no. 2 (1991): 71–87.

21 Bliss, *Banting, A Biography*, 231–97; John Bryden, *Deadly Allies: Canada's Secret War, 1937–1947* (Toronto: McClelland and Stewart 1989), 4–79.

22 Interview with Drs Barbara and C.J. Wyatt, 11 February 1995, by author; Barr and Rossiter, "James Bertram Collip, 1892–1965," 249.

23 Barr and Rossiter, "James Bertram Collip, 1892–1965," 249.

24 Proceedings of the Seventh Meeting of the Associate Committee on Medical Research, 23 October 1941, Records Office, NRC; Gladys L. Hobby, *Penicillin: Meeting the Challenge* (New Haven: Yale University Press 1985), 210–11.

25 R.L. Noble, "Memories of James Bertram Collip," 1362; G.H. Ettinger, *History of the Associate Committee on Medical Research* (Ottawa: National Research Council 1946), 12–24; Harry M. Marks, "Cortisone, 1949: A Year in the Political Life of a Drug," *Bulletin of the History of Medicine* 66 (1992): 419–39.

26 Ettinger, *History of the Associate Committee*, 25–38.

27 Bryden, *Deadly Allies*, 80–133.

28 C.J. Mackenzie to F.G. McIntosh, 19 October 1965, "Library" file, Collip Correspondence, Regional Collection, UWO.

29 Romano, "The Associate Committees," 72; Ettinger, *History of the Associate Committee*, app.

30 Proceedings of a Special Meeting of the Associate Committee on Medical Research, 18 March 1944, Records Office, NRC; interview with Harold

Ettinger, c. 1970, by Robert Noble; Elise A. Corbet, *Frontiers of Medicine*, 173.

31 Proceedings of the Sixteenth Meeting of the Associate Committee on Medical Research, 30 October 1945, 11–13, Records Office, NRC.

32 Barr and Rossiter, "James Bertram Collip, 1892–1965," 250.

33 Ettinger, "Medical Research," 332; Stewart, "Reminiscences," 472.

34 Ray Farquharson to J.B. Collip, 19 November 1954, Proceedings of the Nineteenth Meeting of the Advisory Committee on Medical Research – Division of Medical Research, 3–4 March 1955, app. E, Records Office, NRC.

35 Proceedings of the Seventh Meeting of the Executive of the Advisory Committee on Medical Research, 18 December 1948, 3–6, Records Office, NRC; Ettinger, "Medical Research," 327–8; interview with Robert Noble, Vancouver, B.C., 5 June 1990, by author, notes.

36 Shelley McKellar, "Failed Venture: Gordon Murray and the W.P. Caven Memorial Research Foundation, 1949–74," *Canadian Bulletin of Medical History* 18, no. 2 (2001): 241–75; idem, "The Career of Gordon Murray: Patterns of Change in Mid-Twentieth Century Medicine in Canada" (PHD thesis, University of Toronto, 1999), 163–78.

37 Ettinger, "Medical Research," 321–4.

38 J.B Collip to C.J. Mackenzie, 6 October 1951, Proceedings of the Twelfth Meeting of the Advisory Committee on Medical Research – Division of Medical Research, 31 October 1951, app. A, Records Office, NRC.

39 Harris, *History of Higher Education*, 563–4.

40 Stewart, "Reminiscences," 472.

41 Ibid.

42 Ray Farquharson to J.B. Collip, 19 November 1954, Proceedings of the Nineteenth Meeting of the Advisory Committee on Medical Research – Division of Medical Research, 3–4 March 1955, app. E, Records Office, NRC.

43 Proceedings of the Eighth Meeting of the Advisory Committee on Medical Research – Division of Medical Research, 28 November 1949, 4–5, Records Office, NRC; Ettinger, "Medical Research," 324–6.

44 Interview with Harold Ettinger, c. 1970, by Robert Noble; Stewart, "Reminiscences," 473.

45 Interview with Harold Ettinger, c. 1970, by Robert Noble. Ettinger and Noble say that Collip was upset about the abrupt manner in which he was asked to resign from the NRC [when he reached retirement age?] and suggest that there were feelings of incompatibility between Collip and Steacie.

46 Ettinger, "Origins of Support," 474; Special Committee Appointed to Review Extramural Support of Medical Research by the Government of Canada, *Report to the Honourable Gordon Churchill, Chairman, the Committee of the Privy Council on Scientific and Industrial Research*, 12 November 1959 (Ottawa, 1959), 5–6.

47 *Report to the Honourable Gordon Churchill*, 9–10.
48 Ibid., 26.
49 Ibid., 31.
50 C.J. Mackenzie to F.G. MacIntosh, 19 October 1965, "Library" file, Collip Correspondence, Regional Collection, UWO.

CHAPTER EIGHT

1 C.J. Mackenzie to F.G. MacIntosh, 19 October 1965, "Library" file, Collip Correspondence, Regional Collection, UWO.
2 Much of the following is derived from Barr and Rossiter, "James Bertram Collip, 1892–1965," 235–67; interview with Kenneth Carroll, 30 July 1991, by author.
3 Interview with Drs Barbara and C.J. Wyatt, 11 February 1995, by author; interview with K.K. Carroll, 30 July 1991, by author; interview with A.E. Neufeld, 18 October 1993, by author; interview with Robert Macbeth, 22 May 1991, by author; interview with A.C. Wallace, 18 October 1993, by author.
4 Interview with Harold Ettinger, c. 1970, by Robert Noble; interview with K.K. Carroll, 30 July 1991, by author; interview with A.C. Wallace, 18 October 1993, by author; interview with Robert Cleghorn, 27 June 1991, by author; interview with Robert Macbeth, 22 May 1991, by author.
5 Interview with K.K. Carroll, 30 July 1991, by author. A patent was taken out on the procedure for isolating vinblastine and offered to the National Cancer Institute (NCI) and the Medical Research Council of Canada – the two granting bodies that had funded the research – in accordance with NCI and MRC regulations. When neither body chose to take up the patent, it was given to the UWO to administer. Robert L. Noble, "The Discovery of the Vinca Alkaloids – Chemotherapeutic Agents against Cancer," *Biochemistry and Cell Biology* 68 (1990): 1344–51.
6 Interview with Drs Barbara and C.J. Wyatt, 11 February 1995, by author; interview with Harold Ettinger, c. 1970, by Robert Noble.

CONCLUSION

1 Yves Gingras, *Physics and the Rise of Scientific Research in Canada* (Montreal & Kingston: McGill-Queen's University Press 1991), 3–8.
2 Michael Bliss, "The Aetiology of the Discovery of Insulin," in *Health, Disease and Medicine: Essays in Canadian History*, ed. Charles G. Roland (Toronto: Hannah Institute for the History of Medicine 1984), 338; Sandra F. McRae, "The 'Scientific Spirit' in Medicine at the UT, 1880–1910" (PhD thesis, UT, 1987).

3 The structure of the institute was more important in clinical research through such entities as the Hospital for Sick Children Research Institute (1918), the Montreal Neurological Institute (1932), the Allan Memorial Institute of Psychiatry (1944), the McGill-Montreal General Hospital Research Institute (1945), and the National Cancer Institute (1947).

4 Owen Dyer, "University Accused of Violating Academic Freedom to Safeguard Funding from Drug Companies," *British Medical Journal* 323 (15 September 2001): 591; "Academic Freedom in Jeopardy at Toronto," *Canadian Association of University Teachers Bulletin (Online)* 48, no. 5 (2001), <http://www.caut.ca/english/bulletin/2001_may/default.asp>, May 2001.

5 "Report Vindicates Dr. Nancy Olivieri," *CAUT Bulletin Online* 48, no. 9 (November 2001), <http://www.caut.ca/english/bulletin/2001_nov/default.asp>, November 2001.

Bibliography

MANUSCRIPT SOURCES

Fuller Albright Papers, Francis A. Countway Library, Harvard Medical School.

Associate Committee on Medical Research and Division of Medical Research records, Records Office, National Research Council (Canada).

Frederick Grant Banting Papers, Canada Institute for Scientific and Technical Information.

Walter Bradford Cannon Papers, Francis Countway Library of Medicine, Harvard Medical School.

Cardarelli, Nate. "Dr. Adolph Hanson and Karkinolysin." Unpublished typewritten manuscript, January 1986.

Cardarelli, Nate F., and Bernadette M. Cardarelli. "Thymic Extract (Hanson): An Old Controversy Revisited." Unpublished typewritten manuscript.

James Bertram Collip Papers, MS Collection 269, Fisher Rare Books Library, University of Toronto.

James Bertram Collip Papers and Correspondence, Regional Collection, University of Western Ontario.

DME Fellowship cards, Rockefeller Archive Center.

Orville Frederick Denstedt Papers, McGill University Archives.

Herbert McLean Evans Papers, University of California, Berkeley Archives.

Faculty of Medicine records, McGill University Archives.

Adolph Melanchton Hanson Papers, Owen Wangensteen Historical Library of Biology and Medicine, University of Minnesota.

A.B. Hunstman Papers, University of Toronto Archives.

C.N.H. Long Papers, Library of the American Philosophical Society.

James B. Murphy Papers, Library of the American Philosophical Society.
President's Papers, Medical Research, Regional Collection, University of Western Ontario.
Principal's Papers, McGill University Archives.
Report of the work, B.C. Biological Station, Departure Bay, Pacific Biological Station Archives.
Rockefeller Foundation records, Rockefeller Archive Center.
David Landsborough Thomson Papers, McGill University Archives.
Henry Marshall Tory Papers, University of Alberta Archives.
William Rowan Papers, University of Alberta Archives.

INTERVIEWS

Beer, Charles T. Interview by author, 4 June 1991, Vancouver, B.C. Notes, held by author.
Campbell, Walter. Interview by Robert L. Noble, c. 1970. Copy of original tape recording owned by R.L. Noble, held by author.
Carroll, Kenneth K. Interview by author, 30 July 1991, London, Ont. Tape recording, held by author.
Cleghorn, Robert Allen. Interview by author, 27 June 1991, Toronto, Ont. Tape recording, held by author.
Ettinger, Harold. Interview by Robert L. Noble, c. 1970. Copy of original tape recording owned by R.L. Noble, held by author.
Macbeth, Robert A. Interview by author, 22 May 1991. Tape recording, held by author.
Neufeld, A.E. Interview by author, 18 October 1993, London, Ont. Tape recording, held by author.
Noble, Robert L. Interview by author, 4–5 June 1990, Vancouver, B.C. Notes, held by author.
Scott, John, Mrs Scott, Jack Collip, Barbara Wyatt, Rube Sandin, Bruce Collier, and Ralph Shaner. Interview by Michael Bliss, 4 October 1980, Edmonton, Alta. Notes, held by Michael Bliss.
Wallace, A.C. Interview by author, 18 October 1993, London, Ont. Tape recording, held by author.
Wyatt, Barbara, and C.J. Wyatt. Interview by author, 11 February 1995, Rome, Ga. Tape recording and notes, held by author.

PUBLISHED SOURCES

"Academic Freedom in Jeopardy at Toronto." *Canadian Association of University Teachers Bulletin (Online)* 48, no. 5 (2001) <http: //www.caut.ca/english/bulletin/2001_may/default.asp>, May 2001.

Ainley, Marianne Gosztonyi. *Restless Energy: A Biography of William Rowan, 1891–1957*. Montreal: Véhicule Press 1993.

–, ed. *Despite the Odds: Essays on Canadian Women and Science*. Montreal: Véhicule Press 1989.

Albright, Fuller, and Read Ellsworth. *Uncharted Seas*, edited by D. Lynn Loriaux. Portland, Oreg.: Kalmia Press 1990.

Allen, Garland. *Life Science in the Twentieth Century*. Cambridge: Cambridge University Press 1975.

Amoroso, E.C., and G.W. Corner. "Herbert McLean Evans." *Biographical Memoirs of Fellows of the Royal Society* 18 (1972): 83–186.

Anderson, E.M., and J.B. Collip. "Thyreotropic Hormone of Anterior Pituitary." *Proceedings of the Society for Experimental Biology and Medicine* 30 (1933): 680–3.

Anderson, Evelyn M., and J.B. Collip. "Preparation and Properties of an Anti-thyrotropic Substance." *Lancet* 226 (1934): 784–6.

– "Studies on the Physiology of the Thyreotropic Hormone of the Anterior Pituitary." *Journal of Physiology* 82 (1934): 11–25.

Apfel, Roberta J., and Susan M. Fisher. *To Do No Harm: DES and the Dilemmas of Modern Medicine*. New Haven, Conn.: Yale University Press 1984.

Apple, Rima D. "Patenting University Research: Harry Steenbock and the Wisconsin Alumni Research Foundation." *Isis* 80 (1989): 375–94.

Aronson, Naomi. "The Discovery of Resistance: Historical Accounts and Scientific Careers." *Isis* 77 (1986): 630–46.

Aurbach, G.D. "Purification of Parathyroid Hormone." In *The Parathyroids: Proceedings of a Symposium on Advances in Parathyroid Research*, ed. Roy O. Greep and Roy V. Talmage, 51–9. Springfield, Ill.: Charles C. Thomas 1961.

Austoker, Joan, and Linda Bryder, eds. *Historical Perspectives on the Role of the MRC*. Oxford: Oxford University Press 1989.

Avery, Donald. *The Science of War: Canadian Scientists and Allied Military Technology during the Second World War*. Toronto: University of Toronto Press 1998.

Bachman, Carl, J.B. Collip, and Hans Selye. "Anti-Gonadotropic Substances." *Proceedings of the Society for Experimental Biology and Medicine* 32 (1934): 544–7.

Banting, Frederick Grant, and C.B. Stewart, *Survey of Facilities for Medical Research in Canada*. Ottawa: National Research Council 1939.

Banting, Frederick Grant, C.H. Best, J.B. Collip, and J.J.R. Macleod. "The Preparation of Pancreatic Extracts Containing Insulin." *Transactions of the Royal Society of Canada* 16, section 5 (1922): 27–9.

– "The Effect of Insulin on the Excretion of Ketone Bodies by the Diabetic Dog." *Transactions of the Royal Society of Canada* 16, section 5 (1922): 43–4.

Banting, Frederick Grant, C.H. Best, J.B. Collip, J.J.R. Macleod, and E.C. Noble. "The Effect of Insulin on Normal Rabbits and on Rabbits Rendered Hyperglycaemic in Various Ways." *Transactions of the Royal Society of Canada* 16, section 5 (1922): 31–3.

- "The Effect of Insulin on the Percentage Amounts of Fat and Glycogen in the Liver and Other Organs of Diabetic Animals." *Transactions of the Royal Society of Canada* 16, section 5 (1922): 39–42.

Banting, Frederick Grant, C.H. Best, J.B. Collip, J. Hepburn, and J.J.R. Macleod. "The Effect Produced on the Respiratory Quotient by Injections of Insulin." *Transactions of the Royal Society of Canada* 16, section 5 (1922): 35–7.

Barr, Murray Llewellyn. *A Century of Medicine at Western*. London, Ont.: University of Western Ontario 1977.

Barr, M.L., and R.J. Rossiter. "James Bertram Collip, 1892–1965." *Biographical Memoirs of Fellows of the Royal Society* 19 (1973): 235–67.

Bell, Susan E. "A New Model of Medical Technology Development: A Case Study of DES." *Research in the Sociology of Health Care* 4 (1986): 1–32.

- "Changing Ideas: The Medicalization of Menopause." *Social Science and Medicine* 24 (1987): 535–42.

Benison, Saul, A. Clifford Barger, and Elin L. Wolfe. *Walter B. Cannon: The Life and Times of a Young Scientist*. Cambridge, Mass., and London: Belknap Press 1987.

Bensley, Edward H., ed. *McGill Medical Luminaries*. Montreal: Osler Library 1990.

Berliner, Howard S. *A System of Scientific Medicine: Philanthropic Foundations in the Flexner Era*. New York and London: Tavistock Publications 1985.

Berman, Louis. "A Crystalline Substance from the Parathyroid Glands That Influences the Calcium Content of the Blood." *Proceedings of the Society for Experimental Biology and Medicine* 21 (1923–24): 464.

- "Separation of an Internal Secretion of the Parathyroid Glands." *Journal of Laboratory and Clinical Medicine* 11 (1925–26): 412–13.

- "Priority in the Isolation of Parathyroid Hormone." *Journal of the American Medical Association* 89 (1927): 310–11.

- "The Effect of a Protein-Free Acid-Alcohol Extract of the Parathyroid Glands upon the Calcium Content of the Blood and the Electrical Irritability of the Nerves of Parathyroidectomized and Normal Animals." *American Journal of Physiology* 57 (1935–36): 358–65.

Bissell, Claude. *The Young Vincent Massey*. Toronto: University of Toronto Press 1981.

Bliss, Michael. *The Discovery of Insulin*. Toronto: McClelland and Stewart 1982.

– "The Aetiology of the Discovery of Insulin." In *Health, Disease and Medicine: Essays in Canadian History*, edited by Charles G. Roland, 333–46. Toronto: Hannah Institute for the History of Medicine 1984.

– *Banting, A Biography*. Toronto: McClelland and Stewart 1984.

– *Northern Enterprise*. Toronto: McClelland and Stewart 1987.

– "J.B. Collip: A Forgotten Member of the Insulin Team: In *Essays in the History of Canadian Medicine*, edited by Wendy Mitchinson and Janice Dickin McGinnis, 110–25. Toronto: McClelland and Stewart 1988.

– "Rewriting Medical History: Charles Best and the Banting and Best Myth." *Journal of the History of Medicine and Allied Sciences* 48, no. 3 (1993): 253–74.

Borell, Merriley. "Brown-Séquard's Organotherapy and Its Appearance in America at the End of the Nineteenth Century." *Bulletin of the History of Medicine* 50 (1976): 309–20.

– "Origins of the Hormone Concept: Internal Secretions and Physiological Research, 1889–1905." PhD dissertation, Yale University, 1976.

– "Organotherapy, British Physiology and Discovery of the Internal Secretions." *Journal of the History of Biology* 9 (1976): 235–68.

– "Setting the Standards for a New Science: Edward Schäfer and Endocrinology." *Medical History* 22 (1978): 282–90.

– "Organotherapy and the Emergence of Reproductive Endocrinology." *Journal of the History of Biology* 18 (1985): 1–30.

– "Biologists and the Promotion of Birth Control Research, 1919–1938." *Journal of the History of Biology* 20 (1987): 51–87.

Brown, E. Richard. *Rockefeller Medicine Men: Medicine and Capitalism in America*. Berkeley and Los Angeles: University of California Press 1979.

Browne, J.S.L., and O.F. Denstedt. "James Bertram Collip (1892–1965)." *Endocrinology* 79 (1966): 225–8.

Bryden, John. *Deadly Allies: Canada's Secret War 1937–1947*. Toronto: McClelland and Stewart 1989.

Bullough, Vern L. "Katharine Bemont Davis, Sex Research and the Rockefeller Foundation." *Bulletin of the History of Medicine* 62 (1988): 74–89.

Burrows, Robert. "Variations Produced in Bones of Growing Rats by Parathyroid Extracts." *American Journal of Anatomy* 62 (1938): 237–90.

Campbell, A.D., and J.B. Collip. "On the Clinical Use of the Ovary Stimulating Hormone of the Placenta: Preliminary Report." *Canadian Medical Association Journal* 22 (1930): 219–20.

Canadian Who's Who, 1936–37. Toronto: Times Publishing Co., 1937. S.v. "Macaulay, Thomas Bassett."

Chartrand, Luc, Raymond Duchesne, and Yves Gingras. *Histoire des sciences au Québec*. Montreal: Boréal 1987.

Chittenden, Russell H. *The Development of Physiological Chemistry in the United States*. New York: Chemical Catalog 1930.

The City of the Bay: Belleville and Her Industries. Souvenir Industrial Number of the *Daily Intelligencer*, 1909.

Clark, E.P., and J.B. Collip. "A Study of the Tisdall Method for the Determination of Blood Serum Calcium with a Suggested Modification." *Journal of Biological Chemistry* 63 (1925): 461–4.

Clarke, Adele E. "Emergence of the Reproductive Research Enterprise: A Sociology of Biological, Medical and Agricultural Science in the United States." PhD dissertation, University of California, San Francisco, 1985.

– "Research Materials and Reproductive Science in the United States, 1910–1940." In *Physiology in the American Context, 1850–1940*, edited by Gerald L. Geison. Bethesda, Md.: American Physiological Society 1987.

– "Controversy and the Development of Reproductive Sciences." *Social Problems* 37 (1990): 18–37.

– "Women's Health: Life-Cycle Issues." In *Women, Health and Medicine in America: A Historical Handbook*, edited by Rima D. Apple, 3–39. New Brunswick, N.J.: Rutgers University Press 1990.

Clow, Barbara. "Mahlon William Locke: 'Toe-twister.'" *Canadian Bulletin of Medical History* 9 (1992): 17–39.

Coleman, William. *Biology in the Nineteenth Century: Problems in Form, Function and Transformation*. New York: Wiley 1971.

Coleman, William, and Frederic L. Holmes, eds. *The Investigative Enterprise: Experimental Physiology in 19th Century Medicine*. Berkeley: University of California Press 1988.

Collip, James Bertram. "Some Observations on the Structure and Microchemistry of Nerve Cells." MA thesis, University of Toronto, 1913.

– "Mind and the Cerebral Mechanism." *Trinity University Review* 26, no. 4 (January 1914): 79–81.

– "Further Evidence of an Organic Evolution of Life." *Trinity University Review* 27, no. 4 (January 1915): 81–2.

– "Internal Secretions." *Canadian Medical Association Journal* 6 (1916): 1063–9.

– "Antagonism of Inhibitory Action of Adrenalin and Depression of Cardiac Vagus by a Constituent of Certain Tissue Extracts." *American Journal of Physiology* 53 (1920): 343–54.

– "Antagonism of Depressor Action of Small Doses of Adrenalin by Tissue Extracts." *American Journal of Physiology* 53 (1920): 477–82.

– "The Significance of the Calcium-ion in the Cell – Experimental Tetany." *Canadian Medical Association Journal* 10 (1920): 935–7.

– "Effect of Sleep upon the Alkali Reserve of the Plasma." *Journal of Biological Chemistry* 41 (1920): 473–4.

– "Osmotic Pressure of Serum and Erythrocytes in Various Vertebrate Types as Determined by the Cryoscopic Method." *Journal of Biological Chemistry* 42 (1920): 207–12.

– "Effect of Dilution on the Osmotic Pressure and the Electrical Conductivity of Whole Blood, Blood Serum, and Corpuscles." *Journal of Biological Chemistry* 42 (1920): 213–20.

– "Osmotic Pressure of Tissue as Determined by the Cryoscopic Method." *Journal of Biological Chemistry* 42 (1920): 221–6.

– "Maintenance of Osmotic Pressure within the Nucleus." *Journal of Biological Chemistry* 42 (1920): 227–36.

– "The Alkali Reserve of Marine Fish and Invertebrates." *Journal of Biological Chemistry* 44 (1920): 329–44.

– "Studies on Molluscan Celomic Fluid. Effect of Change in Environment on the Carbon Dioxide Content of the Celomic Fluid. Anaerobic Respiration in Mya Arenaria." *Journal of Biological Chemistry* 45 (1920): 23–49.

– *On the Formation of Hydrochloric Acid in the Gastric Tubes of the Vertebrate Stomach.* University of Toronto Studies, Physiological Series, no. 35. Toronto: University of Toronto Press 1920.

– "Reversal of Depressor Action of Small Doses of Adrenalin." *American Journal of Physiology* 55 (1921): 450–4.

– "A Further Study of the Respiratory Processes in Mya Arenaria and Other Marine Mollusca." *Journal of Biological Chemistry* 49 (1921): 297–310.

– "Delayed Manifestation of the Physiological Effects of Insulin Following the Administration of Certain Pancreatic Extracts." *American Journal of Physiology* 63 (1923): 391–2.

– "The Occurrence of Ketone Bodies in the Urine of Normal Rabbits in a Condition of Hypoglycemia Following the Administration of Insulin – A Condition of Acute Acidosis Experimentally Produced." *Journal of Biological Chemistry* 55 (1923): xxxviii–xxxix.

– "The Demonstration of an Insulin-like Substance in the Tissues of the Clam (Mya Arenaria)." *Journal of Biological Chemistry* 55 (1923): xxxix.

– "The Original Method as Used for the Isolation of Insulin in Semipure Form for the Treatment of the First Clinical Cases." *Journal of Biological Chemistry* 55 (1923): xl–xli.

– "The Demonstration of a Hormone in Plant Tissues to Be Known as 'Glucokinin.'" *Proceedings of the Society for Experimental Biology and Medicine* 20 (1923): 321–3.

– "Glucokinin. A New Hormone Present in Plant Tissue. Preliminary Paper." *Journal of Biological Chemistry* 56 (1923): 513–43.

– "Glucokinin. Second Paper." *Journal of Biological Chemistry* 57 (1923): 65–78.

– "Glucokinin. An Apparent Synthesis in the Normal Animal of a Hypoglycemia-producing Principle. Animal passage of the principle." *Journal of Biological Chemistry* 58 (1923): 163–208.

– "Effect of Plant Extracts on Blood Sugar." *Nature* 111 (1923): 571.

- "The Effect of Insulin on the Oxygen Consumption of Certain Marine Fish and Invertebrates." *American Journal of Physiology* 72 (1925): 181–2.
- "Clinical Use of the Parathyroid Hormone." *Canadian Medical Association Journal* 15 (1925): 1158.
- "The Extraction of a Parathyroid Hormone Which Will Prevent or Control Parathyroid Tetany and Which Regulates the Level of Blood Calcium." *Journal of Biological Chemistry* 63 (1925): 395–438.
- "The Internal Secretion of the Parathyroid Glands." *International Clinics* 3 (1925): 77–80.
- "The Internal Secretion of the Parathyroid Glands." *Proceedings of the National Academy of Science* 11 (1925): 484–5.
- "Animal Passage Hypoglycaemia." *Proceedings of the Society for Experimental Biology and Medicine* 24 (1927): 731–2.
- "The Calcium Mobilizing Hormone of the Parathyroid Glands: Chemistry and Physiology." *Journal of the American Medical Association* 88 (19 February 1927): 565–6.
- "The Parathyroid Glands." *The Harvey Lectures* 21 (1927): 113–72.
- "A Non-specific Pressor Principle Derived from a Variety of Tissues." *Journal of Physiology* 66 (1928): 416–30.
- "A Non-specific Pressor Substance." *American Journal of Physiology* 85 (1928): 360–1.
- "A Non-specific Pressor Substance." *Transactions of the Royal Society of Canada* 22 (1928): 181–4.
- "The Ovary Stimulating Hormone of the Placenta." *Nature* 125 (1930): 444.
- "The Ovary-stimulating Hormone of the Placenta: Preliminary Paper." *Canadian Medical Association Journal* 22 (1930): 216.
- "Further Observations on an Ovary-Stimulating Hormone of the Placenta." *Canadian Medical Association Journal* 22 (1930): 761–74.
- "Placental Hormones." *Proceedings of the California Academy of Medicine* 1 (1930): 47.
- "The Interrelationship between the Pituitary Gland, the Ovaries and the Placenta." *Transactions of the Royal Society of Canada* 26, section 5 (1932): 4–5.
- "The Anterior Pituitary Lobe: Fractionation of Active Principle." *Lancet* 224 (1933): 1208–9.
- "Chemistry and Physiology of Anterior Pituitary Hormones." *Transactions of the Congress of American Physicians and Surgeons* 15 (1933): 47–64.
- "Inhibitory Hormones and the Principle of Inverse Response." *Annals of Internal Medicine* 8 (1934): 10–13.
- "Hormones in Relation to Human Behavior." In Harvard Tertcentenary Conference of Arts and Sciences, *Factors Determining Human Behavior.* Cambridge, Mass.: Harvard University Press 1937.

– "Results of Recent Studies on Anterior Pituitary Hormones." *Edinburgh Medical Journal* 45 (1938): 801.

– Demonstration of an Orally Active Medullotrophic Principle in a Primary Extract of Pituitary Tissue." *Canadian Medical Association Journal* 42 (1940): 965–9.

Collip, James Bertram, and Evelyn M. Anderson. "Studies on the Thyrotropic Hormone of the Anterior Pituitary." *Journal of the American Medical Association* 104 (1935): 965–9.

Collip, James Bertram, Evelyn M. Anderson, and D.L. Thomson. "The Adrenotropic Hormone of the Anterior Pituitary Lobe." *Lancet* 225 (1933): 347–8.

Collip, James Bertram, and P.L. Backus. "The Alkali Reserve of the Blood Plasma, Spinal Fluid and Lymph." *American Journal of Physiology* 51 (1920): 551–67.

– "The Effect of Prolonged Hyperpnoea on the Carbon Dioxide Combining Power of the Plasma, the Carbon Dioxide Tension of Alveolar Air and the Excretion of Acid and Basic Phosphate and Ammonia by the Kidney." *American Journal of Physiology* 51 (1920): 568–79.

Collip, James Bertram, J.S.L. Browne, and D.L. Thomson. "The Relation of Emmenin to Other Estrogenic Hormones." *Journal of Biological Chemistry* 97 (1932): xvii–xviii.

Collip, James Bertram, and E.P. Clark. "Further Studies on the Physiolgical Action of a Parathyroid Hormone." *Journal of Biological Chemistry* 64 (1925): 485–507.

– "Further Studies on the Parathyroid Hormone: Second Paper." *Journal of Biological Chemistry* 66 (1925): 133–7.

– "Concerning the Relation of Guanidine to Parathyroid Tetany." *Journal of Biological Chemistry* 67 (1926): 679–87.

Collip, James Bertram, E.P. Clark, and J.W. Scott. "The Effect of a Parathyroid Hormone on Normal Animals." *Journal of Biological Chemistry* 63 (1925): 439–60.

Collip, James Bertram, and D.B. Leitch. "A Case of Tetany Treated with Parathyrin." *Canadian Medical Association Journal* 15 (1925): 59–60.

Collip, James Bertram, Hans Selye, Evelyn M. Anderson, and D.L. Thomson. "Production of Estrus: Relationship between Active Principles of the Placenta and Pregnancy Blood and Urine and those of the Anterior Pituitary." *Journal of the American Medical Association* 101 (1933): 1553.

Collip, James Bertram, H. Selye, and D.L. Thomson. "Beiträge zur Kenntnis der Physiologie des Gehirnanhanges." *Virchows Archiv für Pathologishe Anatomie und Physiologie* 290 (1933): 23–46.

– "Gonad-Stimulating Hormones in Hypophysectomized Animals. *Nature* 131 (1933): 56.

Collip, James Bertram, H. Selye, and J.E. Williamson. "Changes in the Hypophysis and the Ovaries of Rates Chronically Treated with an Anterior Pituitary Extract." *Endocrinology* 23 (1938): 279–84.

Collip, James Bertram, D.L. Thomson, J.S.L. Browne, M.K. McPhail, and J.E. Williamson. "Placental Hormones." *Endocrinology* 15 (1931): 317.

Collip, James Bertram, D.L. Thomson, M.K. McPhail, and J.E. Williamson. "The Anterior-Pituitary-Like Hormone of the Human Placenta." *Canadian Medical Association Journal* 24 (1931): 201–10.

Corbet, Elise A. *Frontiers of Medicine: A History of Medical Education and Research at the University of Alberta*. Edmonton: University of Alberta Press 1990.

Corner, George W. *A History of the Rockefeller Institute, 1901–1953: Origins and Growth*. New York: Rockefeller Institute Press 1964.

Cushing, Harvey. "Disorders of the Pituitary Gland: Retrospective and Prophetic." *Journal of the American Medical Association* 76 (18 June 1921): 1721–6.

Dancocks, Daniel G. *Sir Arthur Currie: A Biography*. Toronto: Methuen 1985.

Directory of the County of Hastings. Belleville, Ont., 1889.

Doern, Gordon Bruce. *Science and Politics in Canada*. Montreal & Kingston: McGill-Queen's University Press 1972.

Dolev, Eran. "A Gland in Search of a Function: The Parathyroid Glands and the Explanations of Tetany 1903–1926." *Journal of the History of Medicine and Allied Sciences* 42 (1987): 186–98.

Dolman, C.E. "Everitt George Dunne Murray, 1890–1964." *Proceedings of the Royal Society of Canada* 3, series 4 (1965): 145–53.

Dyer, Owen. "University Accused of Violating Academic Freedom to Safeguard Funding from Drug Companies." *British Medical Journal* 323 (15 September 2001): 591.

Edelman, David A. *DES/Diethylstilbestrol – New Perspectives*. Lancaster, England: MTP Press 1986.

Edinburgh University Calendar, 1931–32.

Eggleston, Wilfrid. *National Research in Canada: The NRC 1916–1966*. Toronto: Clarke Irwin 1978.

Ellingson, E.O., A.W. Bell, and Adolph M. Hanson. "Experiments with an Active Extract of Parathyroid." *Proceedings of the Society for Experimental Biology and Medicine* 21 (1923–24): 274–5.

Enros, Philip C. "'The Onery Council of Scientific and Industrial Pretence': Universities and the Early NRC's Plans for Industrial Research." *Scientia Canadensis* 15, no. 2 (1991): 41–51.

Ettinger, G.H. *History of the Associate Committee on Medical Research*. Ottawa: National Research Council 1946.

– "Medical Research." In *Royal Commission Studies: A Selection of Essays Prepared for the Royal Commission on National Development in the Arts, Letters, and Sciences*, 317–36. Ottawa: Edmond Cloutier 1951.

– "The Origins of Support for Medical Research in Canada." *Canadian Medical Association Journal* 78 (1958): 471.

Evans, Herbert M. "Present Position of Our Knowledge of Anterior Pituitary Function." *Journal of the American Medical Association* 101 (1933): 425–32.

Fedunkiw, Marianne Stevens. "Dollars and Change: The Effect of Rockefeller Foundation Funding on Canadian Medical Education at the University of Toronto, McGill University, and Dalhousie University." PhD thesis, University of Toronto, 2000.

Feldberg, Georgina. "The Origins of Organized Canadian Medical Research: The National Research Council's Associate Committee on Tuberculosis Research, 1921–1938." *Scientia Canadensis* 15, no. 2 (1991): 53–69.

Flexner, Abraham. *Medical Education in the United States and Canada: A Report to the Carnegie Foundation for the Advancement of Teaching.* New York: Carnegie Foundation for the Advancement of Teaching 1910.

Frost, Stanley Brice. *McGill University for the Advancement of Learning.* Vol. 2, *1895–1971.* Kingston & Montreal: McGill-Queen's University Press 1984.

– *The Man in the Ivory Tower: F. Cyril James of McGill.* Montreal & Kingston: McGill-Queen's University Press 1991.

Fruton, Joseph S. *Molecules and Life: Historical Essays on the Interplay of Chemistry and Biology.* New York: Wiley 1972.

– *Contrasts in Scientific Style: Research Groups in the Chemical and Biochemical Sciences.* Philadelphia: American Philosophical Society 1990.

Geison, Gerald L. *Michael Foster and the Cambridge School of Physiology: The Scientific Enterprise in Victorian Society.* Princeton, N.J.: Princeton University Press 1978.

–, ed. *Physiology in the American Context, 1859–1940. Proceedings of a Conference Held at the National Library of Medicine, Bethesda, Maryland, January 17–18th, 1986.* Bethesda, Md: American Physiological Society 1987.

Gingras, Yves. "Financial Support for Post-graduate Students and the Development of Scientific Research in Canada." In *Youth, University and Canadian Society: Essays in the Social History of Higher Education,* edited by Paul Axelrod and John G. Reid, 301–19. Kingston & Montreal: McGill-Queen's University Press 1989.

– *Physics and the Rise of Scientific Research in Canada.* Montreal & Kingston: McGill-Queen's University Press 1991.

Glick, Thomas F. "On the Diffusion of a New Speciality: Marañon and the 'Crisis' in Endocrinology in Spain." *Journal of the History of Biology* 9 (1976): 287–300.

Goulet, Denis. *Histoire de la Faculté de Medicine de l'Université de Montréal, 1843–1999.* Montreal: VLB 1993.

Greep, Roy O. "Gonadotropins." In *Endocrinology: People and Ideas,* edited by S.M. McCann. Bethesda, Md: American Physiological Society 1988.

Gridgeman, Norman. *Biological Sciences and the National Research Council of Canada*. Waterloo, Ont.: Wilfrid Laurier Press 1979.

Hall, Diana Long. "Biology, Sex Hormones and Sexism in the 1920's." In *Women and Philosophy: Toward a Theory of Liberation*, edited by Carol C. Gould and Marx W. Wartofsky. New York: G.P. Putnam's Sons 1976.

– "The Critic and the Advocate: Contrasting British Views on the State of Endocrinology in the Early 1920's." *Journal of the History of Biology* 9 (1976): 269–85.

Hall, Diana Long, and Thomas Glick. "Endocrinology: A Brief Introduction." *Journal of the History of Biology* 9 (1976): 229–33.

Hankins, Thomas L. "In Defense of Biography: The Use of Biography in the History of Science." *History of Science* 17 (1979): 1–16.

Hanson, Adolph Melanchton. "An Elementary Chemical Study of the Parathyroid Glands of Cattle." *Military Surgeon* 53 (March 1923): 280–4.

– "Notes on the Hydrochloric X of the Bovine Parathyroid." *Military Surgeon* 53 (April 1923): 434.

– "The Hydrochloric X of the Bovine Parathyroid and Its Phosphotungstic Acid Precipitate." *Military Surgeon* 54 (January 1924): 76–81.

– "The Hydrochloric X Sicca: A Parathyroid Preparation for Intramuscular Injection." *Military Surgeon* 54 (February 1924): 218–19.

– "Parathyroid Preparations." *Military Surgeon* 54 (May 1924): 554–60.

– "Experiments with Active Preparations of Parathyroid Other Than That of the Desiccated Gland." *Military Surgeon* 54 (December 1924): 701–18.

– "The Hormone of the Parathyroid Gland – Changes in the Blood Serum Calcium of Thyroparathyroidectomized Dogs Modified by the Bovine Hydrochloric X." *Minnesota Medicine* 8 (May 1925): 283–5.

– "The Hormone of the Parathyroid Gland." *Proceedings of the Society for Experimental Biology and Medicine* 22 (1925): 560–1.

– "The Standardization of Parathyroid Activity." *Journal of the American Medical Association* 90 (10 March 1928): 747–8.

– "Physiology of the Parathyroid." *Journal of the American Medical Association* 105 (13 July 1935): 113–14.

Harris, Robin S. *A History of Higher Education in Canada, 1663–1960*. Toronto: University of Toronto Press 1976.

Hjort, A.M., S.C. Robison, and F.H. Tendick. "An Extract Obtained from the External Bovine Parathyroid Glands Capable of Inducing Hypercalcemia in Normal and Thyreoparathyroprivic Dogs." *Journal of Biological Chemistry* 65 (1925): 117–28.

Hobby, Gladys L. *Penicillin: Meeting the Challenge*. New Haven, Conn.: Yale University Press 1985.

Holmes, Frederic L. "The History of Biochemistry: A Review of the Literature of the Field." *Biochemistry Collections: A Cross-Disciplinary Survey of the Literature* 1, special collections (1981): 7–16.

- "The Fine Structure of Scientific Creativity." *History of Science* 19 (1981): 60–9.
- "Lavoisier and Krebs: The Individual Scientist in the Near and Deeper Past." *Isis* 75 (1984): 131–42.
- *Hans Krebs: The Formation of a Scientific Life, 1900–1933.* Vol. 1. New York and Oxford: Oxford University Press 1991.

Jackson, Mary Percy. Edited and with an introduction by Janice Dickin McGinnis. *Suitable for the Wilds: Letters from Northern Alberta, 1921–1931.* Toronto: University of Toronto Press 1995.

Jarrell, Richard A., and Normal R. Ball, eds. *Science, Technology and Canadian History. The First Conference on the Study of the History of Canadian Science and Technology.* Waterloo, Ont.: Wilfrid Laurier Press 1980.

Jarrell, Richard A., and Yves Gingras, eds. *Building Canadian Science: The Role of the National Research Council.* Ottawa: Canadian Science and Technology Historical Association 1992. Special number of *Scientia Canadensis* 15, no. 2 (1991).

Jarrell, Richard A., and Arnold E. Roos, eds. *Critical Issues in the History of Canadian Science, Technology and Medicine. Second Conference on the History of Canadian Science, Technology and Medicine, Kingston, Ontario, 1981.* Thornhill, Ont.: HSTC Publications 1983.

Keys, David A. "James Bertram Collip." *Canadian Medical Association Journal* 93 (1965): 774–5.

King, E. Christine. *E. W.R. Steacie and Science in Canada.* Toronto: University of Toronto Press 1989.

Kohler, Robert. "The Management of Science: The Experience of Warren Weaver and the Rockefeller Foundation Programme in Molecular Biology." *Minerva* 14 (1976): 279–306.

- *From Medical Chemistry to Biochemistry.* Cambridge: Cambridge University Press 1982.
- *Partners in Science.* Chicago: University of Chicago Press 1991.

Lane-Petter, W. "The Experimental Animal in Research." In *Techniques in Endocrine Research*, edited by Peter Eckstein and Francis Knowles, 149–59. London: Academic Press 1963.

Latour, Bruno, and Steve Woolgar. *Laboratory Life: The Social Construction of Scientific Facts.* Beverley Hills, Calif.: Sage Publications 1979.

Leathem, James H. "The Antihormone Problem in Endocrine Therapy." *Recent Progress in Hormone Research* 4 (1949): 143.

Lederer, Susan E. "Political Animals: The Shaping of Biomedical Research Literature in Twentieth-Century America." *Isis* 83 (1992): 61–79.

Levere, Trevor. "What Is Canadian about Science in Canadian History?" In *Science, Technology and Canadian History*, edited by R.A. Jarrell and N.R. Ball, 14–22. Waterloo, Ont.: Wilfrid Laurier University Press 1980.

Lewis, D. Sclater. *Royal Victoria Hospital, 1887–1947.* Montreal: McGill University Press, 1969.

– "McGill's First Full-Time Dean of Medicine: Dr. 'Charlie' Martin." In *The McGill You Knew: An Anthology of Memories, 1920–1960*, edited by Edgar Andrew Collard. Toronto: Longman Canada 1975.

Li, Alison. "Expansion and Consolidation: The Associate Committee and the Division of Medical Research of the National Research Council, 1938–1959." *Scientia Canadensis* 15, no. 2 (1991): 89–103.

– "J.B. Collip, A.M. Hanson, and the Isolation of the Parathyroid Hormone, or Endocrines and Enterprise." *Journal of the History of Medicine and Allied Sciences* 47, no. 2 (1992): 405–38.

– "Marketing Menopause: Science and the Public Relations of Premarin," in *Women, Health and Nation: Canada and the United States since 1945*, edited by Gina Feldberg, Molly Ladd-Taylor, Alison Li, and Kathryn McPherson. Montreal & Kingston: McGill-Queen's University Press 2003.

Li, Choh Hao, Herbert M. Evans, and Miriam E. Simpson. "Adrenocorticotrophic Hormone." *Journal of Biological Chemistry* 149 (1943): 413–24.

Liebenau, Jonathan. *Medical Science and Medical Industry: The Formation of the American Pharmaceutical Industry*. Baltimore, Md.: Johns Hopkins University Press 1987.

– "The MRC and the Pharmaceutical Industry: The Model of Insulin." In *Historical Perspectives on the Role of the MRC*, edited by Joan Austoker and Linda Bryder, 83–108. Oxford: Oxford University Press 1989.

Lisser, Hans. "The Endocrine Society: First Forty Years (1917–1957)." *Endocrinology* 80 (1967): 5–28.

Long, Diana E. "Physiological Identity of American Sex Researchers between the Two World Wars." In *Physiology in the American Context, 1850–1940*, edited by Gerald L. Geison. Bethesda, Md: American Physiological Society 1987.

– "Moving Reprints: A Historian Looks at Sex Research Publications of the 1930's." *Journal of the History of Medicine and Allied Sciences* 45 (1990): 452–68.

Löwy, Ilana. "Biomedical Research and the Constraints of Medical Practice: James Bumgardner Murphy and the Early Discovery of the Role of Lymphocytes in Immune Reactions." *Bulletin of the History of Medicine* 63 (1989): 356–91.

Ludmerer, Kenneth L. *Learning to Heal: The Development of American Medical Education*. New York: Basic Books, 1985.

Macallum, A.B., and J.B. Collop [Collip]. "A New Substance in Nerve Cells." *Report of the British Association* 83 (1913): 673–4.

MacCallum, William G., and Carl Voegtlin. "On the Relation of Tetany to the Parathyroid Glands and to Calcium Metabolism." *Journal of Experimental Medicine* 11 (1909): 118–51.

McCann, Samuel M. *Endocrinology: People and Ideas*. Bethesda, Md: American Physiological Society 1988.

McCann, William S. "Parathyroid Therapy." *Journal of the American Medical Association* 83 (1924): 1847.

– "Parathyroid Therapy." *Journal of the American Medical Association* 88 (1927): 566–7.

McGill University. *Annual Report, 1928–1948*.

McKellar, Shelley. "The Career of Gordon Murray. Patterns of Change in Mid-Twentieth Century Medicine in Canada." PhD thesis, University of Toronto, 1999.

– "Failed Venture: Gordon Murray and the W.P. Caven Memorial Research Foundation, 1949–74," *Canadian Bulletin of Medical History* 18, no. 2 (2001): 241–75.

McLean, F.C. Keynote address. In *The Parathyroids: Proceedings of a Symposium on Advances in Parathyroid Research*, edited by Roy O. Greep and Roy V. Talmage. Springfield, Ill.: Charles C. Thomas 1961.

McMurray, Dorothy. *Four Principals of McGill: A Memoir 1929–1963*. Montreal: Graduates' Society of McGill University 1974.

McRae, Sandra Frances. "The 'Scientific Spirit' in Medicine at the University of Toronto, 1880–1910." PhD thesis, University of Toronto, 1987.

– "A.B. Macallum and Physiology at the University of Toronto." In *Physiology in the American Context, 1850–1940*, edited by Gerald L. Geison. Bethesda, Md: American Physiological Society 1987.

Marks, Harry M. "Cortisone, 1949: A Year in the Political Life of a Drug." *Bulletin of the History of Medicine* 66 (1992): 419–39.

Marrus, Michael R. *Mr Sam: The Life and Times of Samuel Bronfman*. Viking 1990.

Marx, Walter, Miriam E. Simpson, and Herbert M. Evans. "Bioassay of the Growth Hormone of the Anterior Pituitary." *Endocrinology* 30 (1942): 1–10.

Mazur, Marcia. "Insulin's Forgotten Man." *Diabetes Forecast*, May 1991: 48–9.

Medvei, Victor Cornelius. *A History of Endocrinology*. Lancaster, England: MTP Press 1982.

Merton, R.K. "Priorities in Scientific Discovery: A Chapter in Sociology of Science." *American Sociological Review* 22 (1957): 635–59.

Mika, Nick, and Helma Mika, comp. *Belleville Centenary Flashback*. Belleville, Ont.: Mika 1978.

Mika, Nick, and Helma Mika. *Historic Belleville*. Belleville, Ont.: Mika 1977.

Mitchinson, Wendy, and Janice Dickin McGinnis, eds. *Essays in the History of Canadian Medicine*. Toronto: McClelland and Stewart, 1988.

Munson, Paul L. "Parathyroid Hormone and Calcitonin." In *Endocrinology: People and Ideas*, edited by S.M. McCann. Bethesda, Md: American Physiological Society 1988.

Needham, Joseph, ed. *The Chemistry of Life: Lectures on the History of Biochemistry*. Cambridge: Cambridge University Press 1970.

Neufeld, A.H., and J.B. Collip. "Studies of the Effects of Pituitary Extracts on Carbohydrate and Fat Metabolism." *Endocrinology* 23 (1938): 735–46.

Noble, Robert L. "Memories of James Bertram Collip." *Canadian Medical Association Journal* 93 (1965): 1356–64.

– "The Discovery of the Vinca Alkaloids – Chemotherapeutic against Cancer." *Biochemistry and Cell Biology* 68 (1990): 1344–51.

Noble, Robert L., and J.B. Collip. "A Quantitative Method for the Production of Experimental Traumatic Shock without Haemorrhage in Unanaesthetized Animals." *Quarterly Journal of Experimental Physiology* 13 (1942): 187–99.

Noble, Robert L., C.S. McEuen, and J.B. Collip. "Mammary Tumours Produced in Rats by the Action of Oestrone Tablets." *Canadian Medical Association Journal* 42 (1940): 413–17.

O'Donovan, D.K. "Some Reminiscences of Canadian Endocrinology." *Journal of the Irish Medical Association* 69 (26 June 1976): 298.

O'Donovan, D.K., and J.B. Collip. "The Specific Metabolic Principle of the Pituitary, and Its Relation to the Melanophore Hormone." *Endocrinology* 23 (1938): 718–34.

Oudshoorn, Nelly. "Endocrinologists and the Conceptualization of Sex, 1920–1940." *Journal of the History of Biology* 23 (1990): 162–87.

– "On the Making of Sex Hormones: Research Materials and the Production of Knowledge." *Social Studies of Science* 20 (1990): 5–33.

– "On Measuring Sex Hormones: The Role of Biological Assays in Sexualizing Chemical Substances." *Bulletin of the History of Medicine* 64 (1990): 243–61.

– *Beyond the Natural Body: An Archeology of Sex Hormones.* London & New York: Routledge 1994.

"Panel Discussion on the Pituitary Gland." *Journal of Pediatrics* 8 (1936): 390–401.

"Parathyrin (Collip)." *Endocrinology* 9 (1925): 242.

Parkes, A.S. "The Rise of Reproductive Endocrinology, 1026–1940." In *Sex, Science and Society.* Newcastle-upon-Tyne: Oriel Press 1966.

Paton, D. Noël, and Leonard Findlay. "The Parathyroids: Tetania Parathyreopriva: Its Nature, Cause and Relation to Idiopathic Tetany." Parts 1–4. *Quarterly Journal of Experimental Physiology* 10 (1916): 203–31, 233–42, 243–314, 315–44.

Penfield, Wilder. *The Difficult Art of Giving: The Epic of Alan Gregg.* Boston & Toronto: Little, Brown and Company 1967.

– "Dr. Penfield Describes How His Work at McGill Began." In *The McGill You Knew: An Anthology of Memories 1920–1960*, edited by Edgar Andrew Collard, 147–8. Toronto: Longman Canada 1975.

Pyke, Magus. *The Six Lives of Pyke.* Toronto: J.M. Dent & Sons 1981.

Raacke, I.D. " 'The Die is Cast' – 'I Am Going Home': The Appointment of Herbert McLean Evans as Head of Anatomy at Berkeley." *Journal of the History of Biology* 9 (1976): 301–22.

Rabinowitch, I.M., Marjorie Mountford, D.K. O'Donovan, and J.B. Collip. "Influence of a Specific Hormone of the Pituitary on the Basal Metabolism in Man." *Canadian Medical Association Journal* 40 (1939): 105–7.

Rasmussen, Howard. "Chemistry of Parathyroid Hormone." In *The Parathyroids: Proceedings of a Symposium on Advances in Parathyroid Research*, edited by Roy O. Greep and Roy V. Talmage, 60–9. Springfield, Ill.: Charles C. Thomas 1961.

Rasmussen, Howard, and Lyman C. Craig. "The Parathyroid Polypeptides." *Recent Progress in Hormone Research* 18 (1962): 269–95.

Reed, T.A., ed. *A History of the University of Trinity College, 1852–1952*. Toronto: University of Toronto Press 1952.

"Report Vindicates Dr. Nancy Olivieri." *CAUT Bulletin Online* 48, no. 9 (November 2001) <http://www.caut.ca/english/bulletin/2001_nov/default.asp>, November 2001.

Rockefeller Foundation. *Report*, 1935–1940.

Roland, Charles G., ed. *Health, Disease and Medicine: Essays in Canadian History. Proceedings of the First Hannah Conference on the History of Medicine, McMaster University, June 3–5, 1982*. Toronto: Hannah Institute, 1984.

Romano, Terrie M. "The Associate Committees on Medical Research of the National Research Council and the Second World War." *Scientia Canadensis* 15, no. 2 (1991): 71–87.

Rossiter, Margaret W. *Women Scientists in America: Struggles and Strategies to 1940*. Baltimore and London: Johns Hopkins University Press 1982.

Rossiter, R.J. "James Bertram Collip, 1892–1965." *Proceedings and Transactions of the Royal Society of Canada* 4 (1966): 73–82.

Sawyer, Charles H. "Anterior Pituitary Neural Control Concepts." In *Endocrinology: People and Ideas*, edited by S.M. McCann. Bethesda, Md: American Physiological Society 1988.

Sayers, George, Abraham White, and C.N.H. Long. "Preparation and Properties of Pituitary Adrenotropic Hormone." *Journal of Biological Chemistry* 149 (1943): 425–36.

"The Science Club." *Trinity University Review* 26 (3): 56–57.

Schull, Joseph. *The Century of the Sun*. Toronto: Macmillan 1971.

Schwartz, Theodore B. "Giants with Tunnel Vision: The Albright-Collip Controversy." *Perspectives in Biology and Medicine* 34 (1991): 327–46.

Scott, John W. *The History of the Faculty of Medicine of the University of Alberta, 1913–1963*. Edmonton: University of Alberta 1963.

Selye, Hans. "Adaptation to Estrogen Overdosage: An Acquired Hormone Resistance without Antihormone Formation." *American Journal of Physiology* 30 (1940): 358–64.

– "The General Adaptation Syndrome and the Diseases of Adaptation." *Journal of Clinical Endocrinology* 6 (1946): 117–230.

- *From Dream to Discovery: On Being a Scientist.* New York: McGraw-Hill 1964.
- *The Stress of My Life.* 2nd ed. New York: Van Nostrand Reinhold Co., 1979.

Selye, H., and J.B. Collip. "Fundamental Factors in the Interpretation of Stimuli Influencing Endocrine Glands." *Endocrinology* 20 (1936): 667–72.

Shortt, S.E.D. *Medicine in Canadian Society: Historical Perspectives.* Montreal & Kingston: McGill-Queen's University Press, 1981.

- "Banting, Insulin and the Question of Simultaneous Discovery." *Queen's Quarterly* 89, no. 2 (Summer 1982): 260–73.

Shryock, Richard H. *American Medical Research.* New York: Commonwealth Fund 1947.

Sinding, Christiane. "The History of Resistant Rickets: A Model for Understanding the Growth of Biomedical Knowledge." *Journal of the History of Biology* 22 (1989): 461–95.

- "Clinical Research and Basic Science: The Development of the Concept of End-Organ Resistance to a Hormone." *Journal of the History of Medicine and Allied Sciences* 45 (1990): 198–232.

Solomon, Samuel, and Alan Lawley. "Medical Research in Canada – A History of Accomplishment, A Future of Uncertainty." *Annals of the Royal College of Physicians and Surgeons of Canada* 19, no. 2 (March 1986): 119–22.

Special Committee Appointed to Review Extramural Support of Medical Research by the Government of Canada. *Report to the Honourable Gordon Churchill, Chairman, the Committee of the Privy Council on Scientific and Industrial Research.* Ottawa, 1959.

Standard Dictionary of Canadian Biography, vol. 2: *1875–1937.* S.v. "Macaulay, Robertson."

Stewart, C.B. "Reminiscences on the Founding and Early History of the Medical Research Council of Canada: Part 2." *Annals of the Royal College of Physicians and Surgeons of Canada* 9 (1986): 385–9, 471–3.

Strickland, Stephen P. *Politics, Science and Dread Disease.* Cambridge, Mass.: Harvard University Press 1972.

Swann, John P. *Academic Scientists and the Pharmaceutical Industry: Cooperative Research in Twentieth-Century America.* Baltimore, Md: Johns Hopkins University Press 1987.

"T.B. Macaulay." Obituary. *Globe and Mail,* 4 April 1942.

Terry, Neville. *The Royal Vic: The Story of Montreal's Royal Victoria Hospital 1894–1994.* Montreal & Kingston: McGill-Queen's University Press 1994.

"The Theological Society." *Trinity University Review* 26, no. 5 (February 1914): 107.

Thirty-Five Years in the Pharmaceutical Manufacturing Industry in Canada. Montreal: Ayerst, McKenna & Harrison Ltd 1961.

Thistle, Mel W. *The Inner Ring: The Early History of the National Research Council of Canada*. Toronto: University of Toronto Press 1966.

Thomson, A. Landsborough. *Half a Century of Medical Research*. Vol. 1: *Origins and Policy of the Medical Research Council (UK)*. London: Her Majesty's Stationery Office 1973.

– *Half a Century of Medical Research*. Vol. 2: *The Programme of the Medical Research Council (UK)*. London: Her Majesty's Stationery Office 1975.

Thomson, David Landsborough. "Editorial: Emmenin." *Canadian Medical Association Journal* 32 (1935): 679–80.

– "Dr. James Bertram Collip." *Canadian Journal of Biochemistry and Physiology* 35, suppl. (1957): 3–7.

Thomson, David Landsborough, J.B. Collip, and Hans Selye. "The Antihormones." *Journal of the American Medical Association* 116 (1941): 132–6.

Urquhart, Hugh M. *Arthur Currie: The Biography of a Great Canadian*. Toronto: J.M. Dent & Sons, 1950.

Wailoo, Keith. "'A Disease *Sui Generis*': The Origins of Sickle Cell Anemia and the Emergence of Modern Clinical Research, 1904–1924." *Bulletin of the History of Medicine* 65 (1991): 185–208.

Weiner, Charles. "Patenting and Academic Research: Historical Case Studies." In *Owning Scientific and Technical Information: Value and Ethical Issues*, edited by Vivian Weil and John W. Snapper, 87–109. New Brunswick, N.J.: Rutgers University Press 1989.

"What's a Monkey Gland? It's Largely Buncombe." *Star Weekly* (Toronto), 6 June 1925.

Wiesner, Bertold P., and Norah M. Sheard. *Maternal Behaviour in the Rat*. Edinburgh: Oliver and Boyd 1933.

Winter, L.B., and W. Smith. "On a Possible Relation between the Pancreas and the Parathyroids." *Journal of Physiology* 58 (1923–1924): 108–10.

Yanacopoulo, Andrée. *Hans Selye, ou, La cathédrale du stress*. Montreal: Le Jour 1992.

Young, E. Gordon. *The Development of Biochemistry in Canada*. Toronto: University of Toronto Press 1976.

Index